T0269301

# DEMYSTIFYING THE ENGINEERING PHD

# DEMYSTIFYING THE ENGINEERING PhD

**MONICA F. COX, PHD**
*Department of Engineering Education,*
*The Ohio State University,*
*Columbus, OH, United States*

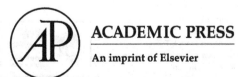

**ACADEMIC PRESS**
An imprint of Elsevier

Academic Press is an imprint of Elsevier
125 London Wall, London EC2Y 5AS, United Kingdom
525 B Street, Suite 1650, San Diego, CA 92101, United States
50 Hampshire Street, 5th Floor, Cambridge, MA 02139, United States
The Boulevard, Langford Lane, Kidlington, Oxford OX5 1GB, United Kingdom

**Notices**
Knowledge and best practice in this field are constantly changing. As new research and experience
broaden our understanding, changes in research methods, professional practices, or medical treatment
may become necessary.

Practitioners and researchers must always rely on their own experience and knowledge in evaluating and
using any information, methods, compounds, or experiments described herein. In using such information
or methods they should be mindful of their own safety and the safety of others, including parties for
whom they have a professional responsibility.

To the fullest extent of the law, neither the Publisher nor the authors, contributors, or editors, assume any
liability for any injury and/or damage to persons or property as a matter of products liability, negligence
or otherwise, or from any use or operation of any methods, products, instructions, or ideas contained in
the material herein.

**British Library Cataloguing-in-Publication Data**
A catalogue record for this book is available from the British Library

**Library of Congress Cataloging-in-Publication Data**
A catalog record for this book is available from the Library of Congress

ISBN: 978-0-12-801593-3

For Information on all Academic Press publications
visit our website at https://www.elsevier.com/books-and-journals

Publisher: Andre Gerhard Wolff
Acquisition Editor: Mary Preap
Editorial Project Manager: Tracy I. Tufaga
Production Project Manager: Swapna Srinivasan
Cover Designer: Matthew Limbert

Typeset by MPS Limited, Chennai, India

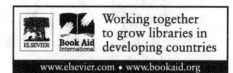

Working together
to grow libraries in
developing countries

www.elsevier.com • www.bookaid.org

# Dedication

I thank God for granting me strength and favor at every point of my academic life. I can't explain how so many doors have opened for me, but I believe that Your hand has guided me to this point, and for that, I am grateful.

To my husband, Ishbah Cox, thank you for your humility and your vision for our family. Every time I have wanted to collapse from life's pressures, you have been there to catch me, to comfort me, and to encourage me to take one more step. Our covenant is real, and we are in this for life.

To my miracle baby, Solomon Cox, thank you for radiating peace from the womb and for comforting me as I finished this book. You represent every promise bestowed on my ancestors. I challenge systems so you will have a better life. Your purpose is bigger than any of us realizes, and I am grateful that God blessed me to be your mother.

To my parents, Jimmy L. and Teresa H. Farmer, thank you for seeing potential in me before I saw it in myself. God gave me a big imagination, and I appreciate your cheering me on even when you didn't fully comprehend the dreams that were in my head. Because of you, I will push myself to achieve big goals until I draw my last breath. I will honor your spirit of service by educating others who want more for themselves.

Thank you to the numerous friends, family, teachers, students, coaches, champions, colleagues, and mentors who have corrected me, lifted me up, cried with me, cheered with me, and prayed for me over my lifetime. I am who I am because of you.

To my editors, Mary Preap and Tracy Tufaga, thanks for your insight and patience as I wrote this book. Seeing this manuscript in print is a dream come true, and I loved sharing this experience with you.

# Contents

## Part III  What Do Engineering PhD Holders Do?          89

### 4.  Characteristics and expectations                        91

## Part IV  How Do You Maximize an Engineering PhD?          123

### 5.  Challenges during transitions and in doctoral education          125

# About the author

Monica F. Cox, PhD, grew up as an single child in a rural southeast Alabama community, where she was raised by her educated parents to persist in the face of personal and professional adversity. She earned degrees in mathematics (Spelman College), industrial engineering (University of Alabama), and leadership and policy studies (Vanderbilt University) debt free and interned at NASA while pursuing her degrees. As a child, she dreamed of traveling to the places she read about, using science to make life better, and entering politics to change the world. Her inquisitive nature contributes to her passion for educating others and sharing what she has learned via her experiences.

She is a professor and inaugural chair of the Department of Engineering Education at The Ohio State University. She is also the director of the International Institute of Engineering Education Assessment (i2e2a) and the CEO of STEMinent LLC, a company that houses educational assessment, professional development, and media offerings. In 2011, she became the first African American female to earn tenure in the College of Engineering at Purdue University. Her research focuses on the use of mixed methodologies to explore significant research questions in undergraduate, graduate, and professional engineering education; explore issues of intersectionality among women, particularly Women of Color (WOC) in engineering; and develop, disseminate, and commercialize reliable and valid assessment tools for use in science, technology, engineering, and mathematics (STEM) education. Dr. Cox has led and collaborated on multidisciplinary projects totaling approximately $16 million, and she has authored over 130 publications.

# Acknowledgments

This material is based in part upon work supported by the National Science Foundation under Grant Number 0747803. Any opinions, findings, and conclusions or recommendations expressed in this material are those of the author(s) and do not necessarily reflect the views of the National Science Foundation. The research described in this book was performed under the Purdue University Institutional Review Board, IRB Protocol #0708005695.

This book would not be possible without the participation of the forty respondents who openly shared the highs and lows of their graduate school and professional experiences and without the guidance of my research project's advisory board.

Thank you to my Ohio State colleagues and research team, especially Dr. Meseret Hailu for copy editing this text, and Dr. Julie Aldridge and Toni Calbert, for encouraging me as I completed this book.

Last but not least, this book reflects the assistance and persistence of my internal and external Purdue University research team (see below) who pushed through recruitment, data collection, and data analyzes to produce numerous publications that have advanced our knowledge about engineering PhD holders. Members of this team have gone on to become faculty and industry employees in the U.S. and around the globe. I hope that the lessons we learned in this study and the "nuggets" presented during our time together will inform your careers and those who follow in your footsteps.

Dr. Benjamin Ahn
Dr. Catherine G.P. Berdanier
Dr. Sara Branch
Dr. Osman Cekic
Shree Frazier
Dr. Jeremi London
Kavitha Ramane
Nikitha Sambamurthy
Anne Tally
Dr. Ana Torres
Tasha Zephirin
Dr. Emily Zhu

## Acknowledgments

# Introduction

According to the Merriam-Webster dictionary, demystify means "to make (something) clear and easy to understand" or "to explain (something) so that it no longer confuses or mystifies someone." Since only a small percentage of people in the world earn doctoral degrees, the definition of the Doctor of Philosophy degree (more commonly referred to as the PhD), the process for obtaining a PhD, and the professional experiences of PhD holders often seem mysterious. Among the questions most often asked to engineers pursuing terminal degrees is "What is a PhD?," "What can you do with an engineering degree?," or "Why should someone pursue a PhD in engineering opposed to a bachelor's or master's degree?" Many of these questions have not been answered in such a way that the average person becomes motivated to pursue graduate education in science, technology, engineering, or mathematics (STEM) or feels comfortable enough to engage in conversations with individuals who possess these degrees.

Although the PhD is understood to be a terminal degree, it does not represent the end of learning. In fact, much like a university commencement, the engineering PhD should be viewed as the certification that new, innovative experiences are about to take place. A person who possesses a PhD in engineering should see this new phase of life as an adventure in which she is viewed as a leader, a technical expert, and an effective communicator. She must be vulnerable enough to admit when she does not have all of the answers and must be humble enough to ask for assistance when needed. These displays of imperfection and teachability among engineering PhD holders might serve as a way to demystify the engineering PhD so that other individuals who do not yet possess the confidence to pursue an undergraduate engineering degree, let alone the PhD, can begin to see this degree as a possibility for themselves.

The majority of engineering PhD holders in the U.S. work in nonacademic environments after graduation (National Science Foundation, 2018). Unfortunately, many engineering doctoral students do not obtain practical, real world, nonacademic experience during their graduate careers, and the majority of engineering faculty have no formal industry experience (National Academy of Engineering, 2005). In addition, many nonacademic employers expect PhD holders to enter their organizations with the capacity to lead teams and to operate as domain experts. To complicate matters even more, industry changes at such a rapid pace that it is likely that an engineering PhD holder might be hired for a job and be expected to work in a completely different area once they begin their employment. Although much is known about demographic trends of engineering PhD holders (National Science Foundation, 2018), less is known about what these PhD holders do, what their experiences are, and how their experiences might inform the next generation of engineering professionals at all levels of the engineering continuum.

Further study of engineering PhD holders is needed given the dearth of literature in graduate engineering education and challenges within doctoral education. Some of the concerns within the U.S. include the following:

- The majority of engineering PhD holders work in non-academic positions (Stephan, Sumell, Black, & Adams, 2004).
- The number of engineering doctoral students interested in pursuing academic jobs is greater than the number of academic jobs available (Fox & Stephan, 2001).
- There is no standard way that many STEM faculty learn to teach; therefore many rely upon their past experiences to develop their pedagogical approaches and techniques (Oleson & Hora, 2014).
- The majority of engineering PhD holders in the U.S. are foreign-born and not permanent residents and/or citizens, a concern across all employment sectors given the U.S.'s need for citizens and permanent residents who might be hired as specialized workers in areas such as security and defense (Cox et al., 2013).
- Traditionally, the PhD offers depth in a particular content area, not breadth. Industry is particularly interested in PhD graduates who demonstrate technical proficiency and transferable professional skills (Akay, 2008; Watson & Lyons, 2011).
- Few, if any policies focus on long-term funding to promote PhD and graduate research in science and engineering (Nemeth, 2014).
- There is no standard accreditation for U.S. engineering PhD programs, thereby increasing variations in PhD program quality in the U.S. and in assessments of doctoral students' experiences (Nemeth, 2014).

## Book overview

With this book, researchers, practitioners, policymakers, university administrators, undergraduate students, and graduate students may find strategies for transitioning across engineering sectors and careers, and at a minimum, gain insight into diverse engineering work environments. Informed by empirical results in which researchers interviewed 40 engineering professionals working in academia and industry across multiple institution types and companies, this work presents information about what it means to be an engineering PhD holder (e.g., expectations and characteristics) and how an engineering PhD holder should contribute to the STEM workforce in knowledge creation, knowledge preservation, and knowledge dissemination.

This book provides insights about *what* PhD holders do and *how* they do what they do to succeed in their jobs. Responses are provided for three points in the life of an engineering PhD holder- the period before pursuing the PhD (i.e., pre-doctoral), the period during which the engineering PhD is being pursued (doctoral), and the period after earning the engineering PhD (postdoctoral). As such, interviewees offered their perceptions about what motivated them to pursue the degree, discussed their daily experiences as engineering PhD holders, and reflected on what they or others might have done differently within their doctoral programs to prepare them for their current jobs. Three overarching research questions guided this study:

1. What are the career paths of respondents from the receipt of their PhDs to their current positions?
2. What does it mean to be an engineering PhD holder?
3. How did graduate school prepare or not prepare respondents for their careers?

Table I.1 lists interview protocol questions aligned with each question and the location of responses in this book.

This book contains four parts with six chapters. Part I, "Why Obtain an Engineering PhD?," explores respondents' motivations for earning engineering PhDs (Chapter 1) and the added value of getting an engineering PhD (Chapter 2). Part II, "What Does it Mean to Be an Engineering Steward?," examines Golde and Walker's (2006) concept of stewardship, or being an engineering scholar, and translates this across three tenets, generation (knowledge discovery), conservation (knowledge preservation), and transformation (knowledge dissemination) (Chapter 3). Part III, "What Do Engineering PhD Holders Do?," examines the (general) characteristics and the (context-specific) expectations of engineering PhD holders across sectors (Chapter 4). Finally, Part IV, "How Do You Maximize an Engineering PhD?," presents challenges respondents

**Table I.1** Research questions, corresponding questions, and location in book.

| Research questions | Protocol questions | Book chapter |
|---|---|---|
| What are the career paths of respondents from the receipt of their PhDs to their current positions? | After looking at the CVs, we will obtain the following information from our respondents if it is missing:<br>• Bachelor's degree discipline and location<br>• Master's degree discipline, location, and research specialization<br>• PhD discipline, location, and research specialization<br>• Most recent job position(s)<br>• (e) Roles, number of years, and location of each position | Introduction |
| | Tell me about the moves you have made in your career and how those moves came about.<br>*(Focus not on just the jobs, but the transition from industry to academia or from academia to industry)* | Chapter 5 |
| | In what ways were you comfortable transitioning from your engineering PhD program to work? Please explain and provide examples. | Chapters 4 and 5 |
| | In what ways were you not comfortable transitioning from your engineering PhD program to work? Please explain and provide examples. | |
| What does it mean to be an engineering PhD? | How did you decide to earn a PhD in engineering?<br>*(Note the influences for the interviewee to obtain the PhD)* | Chapter 1 |
| | Based upon your experiences, is there an added value in gaining a PhD in engineering as opposed to only a Bachelor's or a Master's degree? | Chapter 2 |
| | How would you describe your typical work day (e.g., interactions, work hours)? | Chapter 4 |
| | Within your work environment, what is expected of you as an engineering PhD? | Chapter 4 |
| | | Chapter 3 |

*(Continued)*

**Table I.1** (Continued)

| Research questions | Protocol questions | Book chapter |
| --- | --- | --- |
| | How do you apply knowledge in your field to serve others? | |
| | Give an example of when you have created new and unique knowledge in your field. | Chapter 3 |
| | What are the most important knowledge, skills, norms, attributes, ideas, questions, or perspectives that an engineering PhD should possess? | Chapter 4 |
| | Which of those should be commanded in depth? | |
| | (See previous question) Do you believe your PhD studies equipped you with these? Why, or why not? | Chapter 5 |
| | What are some of the knowledge, skills, norms, attributes, ideas, questions, or perspectives an engineering PhD should understand to conduct research that meets accepted standards of rigor and quality in the field of engineering? | Chapter 3 |
| | (See previous question) Do you believe your PhD studies equipped you to do this? Why or why not? | Chapter 5 |
| | What are the knowledge, skills, norms, attributes, ideas, questions, or perspectives engineering PhDs need to communicate with a variety of audiences? | Chapter 3 |
| | Do you believe your PhD studies equipped you with these knowledge and skills? Why or why not? | Chapter 5 |
| How did graduate school prepare or not prepare respondents for their careers? | Do you think that during your engineering doctoral studies you obtained the skills to do your current job? Why or why not? | Chapter 5 |
| | What can be done at the graduate level to ensure that students are acquiring the desired characteristics that you mentioned earlier? | Chapters 5 and 6 |

experienced during doctoral education and career transitions (Chapter 5) and recommendations for students, faculty, professionals, and university administrators (Chapter 6). Appendices include detailed information about characteristics and expectations of engineering PhD holders along with expanded details about engineering PhD trends.

Chapters are organized similarly. Each chapter begins with a quote illustrating general concepts within that chapter. Responses then are synthesized across the four occupational sectors (i.e., academia, industry, academia to industry, or industry to academia) with primary foci on the most recurring responses in each sector. Each chapter concludes with a section titled "So What?" in which I weave together chapter concepts along with recommendations for engineering professionals and students to translate chapter topics into meaningful actions for themselves and for those around them.

## Research study

Responses in this book are informed from curriculum vitae (CVs) and interviews conducted with 40 engineering professionals with PhDs working in academia and industry. The five-year National Science Foundation grant to conduct this work focused on preparing engineering doctoral students for careers in academia and industry (NSF-EEC-#0747803). Study respondents varied with respect to occupational roles, career trajectories, years of experience, engineering discipline, gender, and nationality (Tables I.2–I.5). Participants' motivations for pursuing engineering PhDs and their careers trajectories also varied.

Although the research team initially wanted to classify respondents as either an academic or industry professional, we soon found that career paths and experiences were not linear and therefore did not focus on a single occupational sector. For example, some respondents graduated with their degrees in engineering, worked in academia and then transitioned to industry or worked in industry and transitioned to academia. In addition, other sectors (e.g., government, nonprofit, and entrepreneurial) were not common among respondents. For this reason, respondents were classified in one of four occupational sectors, which will be used to report findings in each chapter.

**Table I.2** Demographics of respondents who have only worked in academia post-PhD (AC).

| Pseudonym | Engineering field | U.S. Undergrad degree | # Yrs since PhD | Most recent position | Institution's Carnegie classification |
|---|---|---|---|---|---|
| Samantha Ayers | Mechanical | Yes | <5 | Assistant Professor | Baccalaureate College-Diverse Fields |
| Mitchell Bentley | Electrical & Computer | Yes | <5 | Assistant Professor | Master's College and University (larger programs) |
| Sheryl Chambers | Chemical | Yes | <5 | Lecturer | Research University (very high research activity) |
| Bill Richards | Aeronautical | Yes | <5 | Assistant Professor | Master's College and University (medium programs) |
| Darnell Baker | Mechanical & Aerospace | No | 5–10 | Assistant Professor | Research University (very high research activity) |
| Mark Heard | Mechanical | Yes | 5–10 | Research Associate, Lecturer | Research University (very high research activity) |
| Sherrie Roberts | Electrical | Yes | 5–10 | Assistant Professor | Master's College and University (smaller programs) |
| Catrina Benson | Electrical & Computer | Yes | 5–10 | Assistant Professor | Special Focus Institutions--Schools of engineering |
| Linda Stephens | Materials Science & Engineering | No | 5–10 | Assistant Professor | Research University (very high research activity) |
| Christopher Roe | Chemical | Yes | 5–10 | Professor | Doctoral/Research University |
| Miranda Chilton | Mechanical | Yes | 10–20 | Lecturer; Outreach Director | Doctoral/Research University |
| Kevin Magee | Mechanical | Yes | 10–20 | Professor | Master's College and University (larger programs) |
| Juan Cooke | Electrical | Yes | 10–20 | V.P. of Higher Education Policy | Doctoral/Research University |

*(Continued)*

**Table I.2** (Continued)

| Pseudonym | Engineering field | U.S. Undergrad degree | # Yrs since PhD | Most recent position | Institution's Carnegie classification |
|---|---|---|---|---|---|
| Craig Daniels | Biomedical | Yes | 10–20 | Adjunct Assistant Professor | Research Laboratory (non–Carnegie) |
| Stephanie Stahl | Chemical | Yes | 10–20 | Associate Professor | Research University (very high research activity) |
| George Murray | Electrical & Computer | Yes | > 20 | Professor & Department Chair | Research University (very high research activity) |
| Adam Greene | Theoretical & Applied Mechanics | Yes | > 20 | Distinguished Professor | Research University (very high research activity) |

**Table I.3** Demographics of respondents who have only worked in industry post-PhD (IN).

| Pseudonym | Engineering field | U.S. undergrad degree | # Yrs since PhD | Recent position | Company's classification |
|---|---|---|---|---|---|
| Gino Braxton | Industrial | Yes | 10 to 20 | Senior Manager | Mail, package, and freight delivery (ranked between 50 and 100) |
| Julius Kimmel | Chemical | Yes | > 20 | Director, Research and Development | Chemicals (ranked between 201 and 250) |
| Benjamin Kinder | Mechanical | No | 5 to 10 | Mechanical Engineer | Household and personal products (ranked between 101 and 150) |
| Stewart Oglesby | Chemical | No | < 5 | Mechanical Engineer | Household and personal products (ranked between 101 and 150) |
| Ronald Perkins | Industrial | Yes | < 5 | Professional Training Director | Aerospace and defense |
| Arlene Petit | Mechanical | Yes | < 5 | Systems Design Engineer | Ranked outside Fortune 500 classification |
| Nicholas Poole | Electrical | Yes | < 5 | Software Engineer | Internet services and retailing (ranked between 50 and 100) |
| Ginnefer Rankin | Biomedical | Yes | < 5 | Scientist | Household and personal products (ranked between 101 and 150) |
| Bradley Simmons | Chemical | Yes | > 20 | Director, Process Engineering | Network and other communications equipment (ranked between 301 and 350) |
| Nadine Vinson | Chemical | Yes | 5 to 10 | Engineer Associate | Petroleum refining (ranked between 1 and 50) |

1. Academia (AC)- working only in academia after their engineering PhD (17 respondents) Table I.2
2. Industry (IN)- working only in industry after their engineering PhD (10 respondents) Table I.3
3. Academia to Industry (AC-IN)- working in academia and then transitioning to a career in industry (4 respondents) Table I.4
4. Industry to Academia (IN-AC)- working in industry and then transitioning to a career in academia (9 respondents) Tables I.5

Table I.6 displays information about the distribution of these interviewees across disciplines and sectors. The team made deliberate efforts to interview respondents who obtained PhDs in the disciplines that produced the highest number of engineering PhD recipients in 2010, the year that most interviews were conducted, resulting in the largest number of respondents in chemical engineering, mechanical engineering, and electrical engineering (National Science Foundation, 2018). Disciplines identified within the "other" category include biomedical engineering, materials science and engineering, aerospace engineering, and industrial engineering. Although some respondents' degrees represented more than one discipline, we classified them in the field most aligned with their self-identified areas of technical expertise. Twenty-eight percent of our respondents were women, and 13% were considered to be international students at the time they earned their PhDs.

**Table I.4** Demographics of respondents who worked in academia then industry post-PhD (AC-IN).

| Pseudonym | Engineering field | U.S. undergrad degree | # Yrs since PhD | Recent position | Current company's classification |
|---|---|---|---|---|---|
| Peter Renewable energy | Calloway Electrical | Yes | 10−20 | | Chief Technology Officer technology sector |
| Blake Greiner | Mechanical | Yes | 10−20 | Principal Engineer | Construction and farm machinery (ranked between 51 and 100) |
| Virgil Sharma | Electrical | No | 10−20 | Director | Department of Engineering & Technology |
| Ryan Ziegler | Mechanical | Yes | 10−20 | Engineering Technical Steward | Construction and farm machinery (ranked between 1 and 50) |

**Table 1.5** Demographics of participants who worked in industry then academia post-PhD (IN-AC).

| Pseudonym | Engineering field | U.S. undergrad degree | # Yrs since PhD | Recent position | Current Institution's Carnegie classification |
|---|---|---|---|---|---|
| Roland Bankston | Chemical | Yes | 10–20 | Professor | Research University (very high research activity) |
| Eric Dillard | Materials | Yes | 10–20 | Associate Professor | Research University (very high research activity) |
| Philip Hays | Electrical | Yes | >20 | Professor | Research University (very high research) |
| Reuben Moffit | Chemical | Yes | >20 | Lecturer | Research University (very high research activity) |
| Randall Rice | Chemical | Yes | 5–10 | Postdoctoral Fellow | Master's College and University (larger programs) |
| Terry Sherwood | Chemical | Yes | >20 | Founder Sr. Lecturer | Science Consulting Service & Research University (very high research activity) |
| Shirley Thorne | Electrical & Computer | Yes | 10–20 | Assistant Professor | Research University (very high research activity) |
| Aaron Whitehurst | Electrical & Computer | Yes | >20 | Distinguished Professor | Research University (very high research activity) |
| Mark Winkler | Chemical | Yes | 10–20 | Department Chair | Associate's–Public 4-year Primarily Associate's |

**Table I.6** Distribution of respondents by engineering discipline, sector, and gender.

|  | AC | | IN | | AC-IN | | IN-AC | | Total |
|---|---|---|---|---|---|---|---|---|---|
|  | M | F | M | F | M | F | M | F |  |
| Aerospace | – | – | 2 | – | – | – | – | – | 2 |
| Biomedical | 1 | – | – | 1 | – | – | – | – | 2 |
| Chemical | 1 | 2 | 3 | 2 | – | – | 5 | – | 13 |
| Electrical | 3 | 2 | 1 | – | 2 | – | 2 | 1 | 11 |
| Industrial | – | – | 2 | – | – | – | – | – | 2 |
| Mechanical | 3 | 2 | 1 | – | 2 | – | – | – | 8 |
| Materials | – | 1 | – | – | – | – | 1 | – | 2 |
| Grand Total | 8 | 7 | 9 | 3 | 4 | – | 8 | 1 | 40 |

*Sampling and Recruitment Strategy*- Purposive, criterion sampling, was used to identify potential respondents in this study. The primary criterion for all respondents was that they earned a PhD in engineering from a U.S. institution. Bachelor's and Master's degrees may have been obtained from institutions outside the U.S. and could have been obtained in non-engineering disciplines. A sample of both international PhD recipients (were not U.S. citizens or permanent residents when they earned their PhD) and domestic PhD recipients (were U.S. citizens or permanent residents when they earned their engineering PhD) were included in the sample. All international interviewees obtained their undergraduate degrees outside the U.S., and all U.S.-born interviewees obtained their undergraduate degrees in the U.S.

The sampling parameters were set both by Golde and Walker's (2006) framework and the research questions. The sample was pulled from people with academic and industrial perspectives outside my institution. Academic respondents included engineering PhD holders who worked in a variety of traditional academic settings and in non-tenure and tenure-track positions. Industry respondents included engineering PhD holders who worked in a variety of nonacademic settings and in technical and managerial positions. Over time, the sampling of interviewees moved from an explicit focus on the nationality of the respondents (i.e., international or U.S. citizen or permanent resident) to primary engineering disciplinary placement (e.g., chemical engineering) and work sector placement (e.g., working in an industry job first followed by an academic job).

Respondents were recruited via convenience and snowballing strategies. While convenience strategies produced engineering PhD holders across several engineering disciplines, the snowballing strategy was used to identify engineering PhD holders within the three engineering disciplines in which the most engineering PhD holders obtained industry jobs. Initial recruitment of research respondents occurred via email among faculty at a Midwestern research university. A recruitment email was also distributed to appropriate disciplinary and diversity-related listservs within the American Society for Engineering Education (ASEE) to recruit potential interviewees representing diverse sectors and perspectives.

*Interview Protocol* Each respondent was asked to participate in an hour-long interview. A team of interviewers asked 15 questions that focused on three research questions exploring career paths of engineering PhD holders, what it means to possess an engineering PhD, and graduate preparation for engineering PhD students (Table I.1). Golde and Walker's (2006) stewardship framework was an area of focus since we wanted to frame responses in the context of doctoral education and scholarship. An overview of stewardship and other research studies that have been informed by this framework are presented in greater detail in Chapter 3.

## Data analysis

My research team and I conducted all interviews with four people coding interview transcripts using Atlas.ti qualitative software. Glaser and Strauss' (1967) constant comparative method, in conjunction with open coding, was used to interpret all responses. Excerpts of respondent interviews from each sector (i.e., academia, industry, industry to academia, and academia to industry) were combined into a single transcript that members of the research team used to code the data. Intercoder reliability was above 75% across observers when exploring percent agreement and a k-value of 0.61 was obtained within a second round of coding, resulting in "substantial agreement" (Fleiss, 1971) across observers (London et al., 2014). A codebook containing 301 codes across eleven categories was created using the recommendations of MacQueen, McLellan, Kay, and Milstein (1998). Codes for topics are presented in corresponding chapters and in the appendices.

## References

Akay, A. (2008). A renaissance in engineering PhD education. *European Journal of Engineering Education, 33*(4), 403–413. Available from https://doi.org/10.1080/03043790802253475.

Cox, M. F., Zephirin, T., Sambamurthy, N., Ahn, B., London, J., Cekic, O., . . . Zhu, J. (2013). Curriculum vitae analyses of engineering Ph.D.s working in academia and industry. *International Journal of Engineering Education, 29*, 1205–1221.

Fleiss, J. L. (1971). Measuring nominal scale agreement among many raters. *Psychological Bulletin, 76*, 378−382. Available from https://doi.org/10.1037/h0031619.

Fox, M. F., & Stephan, P. E. (2001). Careers of young scientists: Preferences, prospects and realities by gender and field. *Social Studies of Science, 31*(1), 109122. Available from https://doi.org/10.1177/030631201031001006.

Glaser, B. G., & Strauss, A. L. (1967). *The discovery of grounded theory: Strategies for qualitative research*. Chicago: Aldine Publishing.

Golde, C. M., & Walker, G. E. (2006). *Envisioning the future of doctoral education: Preparing stewards of the discipline, Carnegie essays on the doctorate*. San Francisco, CA: Jossey-Bass.

London, J., Cox, A. M., Ahn, B., Branch, S., Torres-Ayala, A., Zephirin, T., & Zhu, J. (2014). Motivations for pursuing an engineering Ph.D. and perceptions of its added value: A U.S.-based study. *International Journal of Doctoral Studies, 9*, 205−227.

MacQueen, K. M., McLellan, E., Kay, K., & Milstein, B. (1998). Codebook development for team-based qualitative analysis. *CAM Journal, 10*(2), 31−36. Available from https://doi.org/10.1177/1525822 × 980100020301.

National Academy of Engineering. (2005). *Educating the engineer of 2020: Adapting engineering education to the new century*. Washington, DC: The National Academies Press. Available from https://doi.org/10.17226/11338.

National Science Foundation, National Center for Science and Engineering Statistics. 2018. *Doctorate recipients from U.S. Universities: 2017*. Special Report NSF 19-301. Alexandria, VA. Available from https://ncses.nsf.gov/pubs/nsf19301/.

Nemeth http://diverseeducation.com/article/66171/ STEM Researchers: Do We Produce Right Stuff? 2014.

Oleson, A., & Hora, M. T. (2014). Teaching the way they were taught?: Revisiting the sources of teaching knowledge and the role of prior experience in shaping faculty teaching practice. *Higher Education, 68*(1), 29−45.

Stephan, P. E., Sumell, A. J., Black, G. C., & Adams, J. D. (2004). Doctoral education and economic development: The flow of new Ph.D.s to industry. *Economic Development Quarterly, 18*(2), 151−167. Available from https://doi.org/10.1177/0891242403262019.

Watson, J., & Lyons, J. (2011). Aligning academic preparation of engineering Ph.D. Programs with the needs of industry. *International Journal of Engineering Education, 27*, 1394−1411.

# Why obtain an engineering PhD?

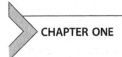

# CHAPTER ONE

# Motivations

*My decisions (to earn an engineering PhD) were not based upon necessarily positive influences as much as negative influences. Undergraduate, I was going to college and most of my experiences there were positive, but even after I finished there I still didn't necessarily want to get my PhD. What really influenced me was my time at [Graduate University]. I was there for about two years, in electrical engineering. And the entire time I was there I never had a female professor and I never had a professor of color. So at [Undergraduate College], most of my professors were African-American females and at [Graduate University] I had none of them. And not only did I not have any mentors that looked like me, or instructors that looked like me, I also felt that their teaching style was not conducive for me to be successful in my learning. So actually as an undergraduate sitting in a classroom, I said, 'I think I can do this better. I think I have a better way. I think that there is a way to give an impression to students of engineering who if they don't look like them, they at least make it look enjoyable and like something they would want to do.' I just feel like the traditional engineering professor is not something that inspires me to want to be an engineer. That's why I decided to get my PhD.*

**Catrina Benson, PhD, Assistant Professor**

How does an engineering PhD holder earn a doctorate? Stories varied across respondents. This chapter provides motivations for pursuing an engineering PhD as told in the voices of people interviewed for this study. Throughout this chapter, motivation is referred to as the reasons that respondents pursued a PhD, including: personal interests, influences from others, and academic-related factors. Findings also explored what motivated respondents to persevere in their pursuit of their degrees, even during hard times. I also present advice for others considering the pursuit of the PhD.

Open-coded responses from interviewees resulted in fourteen occurrences (London et al., 2014). Asset-oriented reasons for pursuing an engineering PhD included:

*Demystifying the Engineering PhD.*
DOI: https://doi.org/10.1016/B978-0-12-801593-3.00001-3

- Exposure to graduate education opportunities (e.g., attending a conference or professional development workshop)
- Interest in a career that requires a PhD (e.g., working as a tenure-track faculty member)
- Influence of a family member
- Encouragement from mentors such as peers, teachers, and professors
- Trends that called for advanced degrees
- Desire to do scientific work
- Opportunity to enter the academic profession
- Commitment to research in general
- Fascination with something associated with one's technical area but not research (e.g., teaching)
- Passion for one's particular technical subject/ topic of interest (e.g., operations research within industrial engineering)
- Personal interest (e.g., going abroad, being challenged intellectually)
- Prior success in graduate school (e.g., engaging in research as a Master's student or passing a qualifying exam), and
- Funding to attend graduate school

Although the majority of the codes were asset-based, one negative motivation (i.e., discontent with one's current job), emerged. Such discontent might relate to having a desire to explore a new dimension within one's job.

## Academia respondents

Members of the research team rank ordered respondents' motivations for earning engineering PhDs. Within academia, the seventeen respondents identified their motivations to be the opportunity to go into the academic profession; personal interests; being passionate about something associated with their technical subject, but not research; being influenced by mentors, teachers, and/or professors; having a goal that necessitates a PhD; and being passionate about research. Elaboration of each of these motivations from the perspectives of academic audiences is presented in this section.

### Opportunity to go into the academic profession

Some engineering PhD respondents currently working in academia recognized early in their careers that earning a PhD in engineering offered a way to obtain university jobs and to achieve their goals of becoming college professors. Although many of the engineering PhD holders loved to teach, they realized they had to conduct doctoral-level research to obtain a PhD to teach at the college level, thereby becoming the required credential for them to become faculty members.

Catrina Benson, an Assistant Professor with graduate degrees in electrical engineering, expounded upon her passion for teaching and its connection to her pursuit of a PhD. She noted that as a woman of color in engineering courses, she also wanted to be a role model for future students of color:

> I loved what I did because the whole purpose for me getting my PhD is I wanted to teach, and I wanted to be an engineering professor; not necessarily do research. I wanted to be an engineering educator. I wanted to educate potentially more students who looked like me and repeat after my own kind. I wanted them to see role models that looked like them. I wanted them to see it could be done.

Many of the respondents who eventually earned a PhD developed interest in the degree early in their undergraduate experiences. Mechanical engineer Miranda Chilton, who works at a doctoral/research university, decided to become a professor as a sophomore engineering student taking thermodynamics. Meanwhile, chemical engineering Full Professor Christopher Roe, whose interest in teaching was piqued during his first year of college and who works at a doctoral/research university, "felt at home" when he taught others. To pursue his passion, he knew he needed to get a PhD. The journey was not easy for him, however, resulting in his almost leaving graduate school with only a Master's of Science degree. At one point, he wanted to return to his childhood home. At that point, he "was reminded that I wanted to be a faculty member, so I decided to stick with it." Similarly, Sherrie Roberts, an Assistant Professor of Electrical Engineering working at a Master's College and University, echoed, "I decided to stay on (in graduate school) for a PhD because I wanted to become a professor. I really loved my professors when I was an undergrad, and I knew that was the job that I wanted to do."

Not all academic respondents decided to earn a PhD as undergraduate students. Kevin Magee, a mechanical engineering professor who worked in the automotive industry after getting his undergraduate degree, pursued a PhD after earning his Master's degree. He realized that his career path was limited at the automotive company where he worked. He explained, "You can only go so far as an engineer before you either go into management or needed (an) advanced degree ... I did not want to go to management, so I went the academic direction." Similarly, Mitchell Bentley, an Assistant Professor, decided to earn a PhD several years after working in the automotive industry: "When I was around 26/27 years old, that's when I made the decision that long-term I wanted to go back and get my PhD and into the ranks of academia and leave the electronics industry completely."

## Personal interests

Several academics noted that their PhD pursuits connected to their personal interests, particularly their desires to help others in the future. Catrina Benson spoke of her transition from a minority-serving, liberal arts institution as an undergraduate to a larger predominately white institution to pursue her engineering degrees. Her desire to have mentors and instructors who looked like her motivated her to enter the professoriate. Miranda Chilton noted an affinity for helping other undergraduate engineering students comprehend course content:

> When I was a sophomore and taking classes I found it very rewarding because I could help my classmates understand material that they were not able to understand from the lecture that had just been given by the professor. And so, I had a way of explaining it that made sense to them. And they liked that. I found it very rewarding to be able to provide knowledge in an understandable manner.

For both Benson and Chilton, their educational experiences in engineering classrooms motivated their pursuits of engineering PhDs. Sitting in a classroom and seeing how they could make a difference for future students informed their career paths as professors.

Similarly, undergraduate experiences drove Distinguished Professor, Adam Greene, and Christopher Roe, to pursue PhDs. As an undergraduate, Greene enjoyed school and realized he needed more than a Bachelor's degree. For this reason, he aimed to attend graduate school.

Although Roe's undergraduate experience was positive, he wavered somewhat once he entered graduate school:

> Very early on I decided I wanted to do the PhD and wanted to be faculty. And I don't think I doubted that for a minute when I was an undergrad. So, perhaps I doubted it a little bit when I was a grad student.

Adjunct Assistant Professor Craig Daniels perceived that his engineering discipline (biomedical engineering) warranted his earning a PhD given the nature of the work he might pursue:

*I think I always wanted a terminal degree. You know engineering, especially biomedical engineering is particularly sensitive with respect to the kind of work you can do as a Bachelor's or Master's level engineer. Especially when it comes to medical devices, you know, they want that PhD for liability purposes. So, unlike a civil engineer or a mechanical engineer who could design a bridge or do whatever, the medical industry is particularly sensitive to having a PhD So, if you really - if you want to do PhD level work, if you want to do really great stuff in bioengineering you have to have a PhD.*

For these respondents, obtaining an engineering PhD connected to both their enjoyment and their disgruntlement of their undergraduate experiences within specific engineering disciplines.

## Being passionate about something other than research

Many of the academic interviewees identified their affinity for something other than their technical area or research as a motivation for earning a PhD. Miranda Chilton, Adam Greene, Sheryl Chambers, and Mitchell Bentley highlighted their love for and interest in teaching. Chilton recalled a graduate education experience that transformed her perspective about the impact of teaching:

*When I went to (Graduate University), they were working with teachers to help them understand engineering to bring it into their classrooms, and I had never even considered an audience besides college students. And as soon as I thought about other audiences, I thought, 'Wow, this is great. I really want to make a difference in the education in this country. And, here's a place I can do it.*

Greene also discovered a love for teaching after receiving a fellowship that offered him an option to be a teaching assistant (TA) versus a research assistant (RA). The breadth of experiences as a TA allowed him to see himself as a future faculty member:

*I had a fellowship but then it was to be supplemented with either a TA or an RA. And I guess I decided I wanted to do a TA because I wanted experience making presentations. I wasn't very comfortable with that. And, their TAs actually taught classes. ... So as a TA I actually taught a strength and statics course, did all the lectures. You know, graded all the homework. And then I also taught a strength and materials course. And, that was fun. That was more interesting than I thought it would be ... I enjoyed that. And I thought, well maybe I'd like to do that sometime.*

Chambers' interest in becoming a professor began in high school. Similar to Greene, a teaching assistant experience fortified her interest in teaching. Chambers, a lecturer with a PhD in chemical engineering, reflected:

*When I was doing my undergraduate work at (Undergraduate University) in chemical engineering, I had the opportunity to be a teaching assistant, I think it might have been in my junior year. But I had the opportunity to be a teaching assistant sometime in my upperclassman years for a freshman course. And it was the first experience that I had had really teaching. And, I had the experience of facilitating kind of a lab class -it was kind of like a computer lab class. And I loved it ... I was very passionate about it, and was very rewarding, and I kind of knew at that point that while I did love engineering, and I loved those courses, and I liked the internships I had done, I really loved the teaching. And so that helped make the decision that I wanted to pursue a PhD so that I could teach at the college level.*

Unlike several respondents, Bentley Mitchell, an Assistant Professor of Electrical and Computer Engineering working at a Master's College, said that his affinity for teaching emerged when he worked in industry, which shows that not everyone who eventually displays a passion for teaching has to identify this affinity as a student:

*And a biggest part of my job became working with these employees in my company and teaching them what I felt was the best way to be an engineer and to solve problems. And that's where I really made the decision while I was still working that I wanted to not only get the PhD but go into academia to work with other engineers and teach them.*

For each of the respondents, teaching began as an enjoyable experience that turned into a possible career choice. Chilton's understanding of teaching extended beyond what she knew in the classroom and made her think of a larger impact she could make through instruction. Greene was serendipitously introduced to teaching as a funded teaching assistant, thereby planting a seed for his future career as a professor. Similarly, being a TA served as Chambers' "aha" moment as a future professor. Bentley's interest in teaching peaked in a nonacademic setting in a quest to help engineers in industry become better problem solvers.

International experiences also might inform one's desire to teach. Mark Heard, a mechanical engineering research associate and lecturer, chose to pursue his doctorate after a graduate research advisor offered him an opportunity to obtain an advanced degree at a U.S. university's campus in France:

*After I finished my Master's I...went to work in (City) for a couple of years. And my Master's advisor then called me kind of out of the blue and said that they were doing... sort of the same thing, so (University) has a campus in France.*

*And that's why I spent time there. And he said, you know, we're trying to do degree programs - PhD degree programs through the French campus and we need somebody to help set up that program, and to help set up research, well ultrasonics research lab there too. And so basically that was the other side of it was it allowed me basically the ability to go live in France again for another four years. So that was a non-negligible part of the decision as well.*

## Influenced by mentors, teachers, and/or professors

Personal connections influenced many of the faculty who chose academic careers. Chilton's father was a professor who modeled the faculty lifestyle at a university. Faculty advisors and professors supported Mark Heard, Samantha Ayers, Sherrie Roberts, Juan Cooke, and George Murray. Ayers, a mechanical engineer working as an Assistant Professor at a Baccalaureate College, shared fond memories about an encouraging advisor who told her, "You'd make a good professor one day, and you know, I think you'd be really good going forward and getting your PhD." This advisor connected her to another professor at a west coast university who later became her advisor.

Murray, a Professor and Department Chair, decided to pursue the PhD during his undergraduate and graduate education under the mentorship of two encouraging advisors. While a number of people recognized his potential as an undergraduate, an alumnus at a west coast research university persuaded him to attend his alma mater after Murray worked at a prestigious lab in a fellowship program.

Cooke, a Vice President of Higher Education Policy, attributed his doctoral aspirations to supportive faculty members and from multiple experiences. He participated in a university program in which graduating students could obtain a faculty rank of instructor. Regarding his advisor, he remembered:

*I had the opportunity to have a PhD advisor that was not only well known and an internationally recognized researcher, but also had a strong passion for teaching. So, I was exposed in my PhD studies to many opportunities that allowed me to not only engage in teaching of undergraduate students at that time but also to engage in training programs for high school teachers and so forth.*

Overall, these respondents' experiences demonstrated the importance of positive connections for students who wanted to obtain a PhD.

## Having a goal that necessitates a PhD

For most faculty, earning a PhD was deemed a necessity early in their engineering journeys. While Craig Daniels reported that he always wanted a terminal degree and asserted that not every engineering discipline mandates that someone earn a PhD, he described the medical industry as "particularly sensitive to having a PhD." Since he wanted to "do really great stuff in bioengineering," he pursued a PhD and asserted that "biomedical engineering is particularly sensitive with respect to the kind of work you can do as a Bachelor's or Master's level engineer. Especially when it comes to medical devices ... they want that PhD for liability purposes."

Miranda Chilton, Catrina Benson, and Samantha Ayers explained that a love of teaching motivated them to pursue a PhD. Coupled with that, however, was Chilton's desire to gain industry experience, Benson's desire to become a professor who served as a role model more than her engineering professors were to her, and Ayers' affinity for learning and schoolwork. Chilton wanted to become an engineering professor with practical work experience mirroring the experiences of some of her professors. She explained:

> When I decided I wanted to be a professor, I started studying and observing the other professors that I had. What I learned from my observation was that I felt that those (professors) that had been out and had real work experience were much better instructors and much more interesting to listen to than those that had remained completely in the academic environment and were very theoretical. So I wanted the same advantage. I wanted to give myself every advantage I could to be a great professor. And I felt that work experience would do that. And so that's why I got a job in industry between my Master's and PhD so that I could have the same experiences.

Juan Cooke's focus on becoming a faculty member fueled his pursuit of a PhD in electrical engineering. For him, "There was never any doubt that that's what I wanted to do ... given my career aspiration at the time ... Since I wanted to be a faculty member I had to get a PhD."

Many respondents who worked only in academia were motivated to pursue a PhD because of a love of teaching and because of the influences of others. Although the PhD is a research-oriented degree, the research was not the initial draw for many of them as they thought about pursuing their PhDs. Many realized that earning a PhD was a necessity if they wanted to become professors even if they did not enjoy research.

## Being passionate about research

Academicians also referred to being passionate about research. Mark Heard noted that research is a big part of earning a PhD and that a graduate student needs to have some love for research during a doctoral experience. Both Kevin Magee and Juan Cooke recalled that their love of teaching and research motivated them to earn an engineering PhD. Cooke wanted to remain at his childhood home to work, although there were limited job opportunities available to him there. For that reason:

*The only path that I had career-wise that would allow me to stay in (Cooke's childhood home) and do research at that time was to get a PhD and come back to the university as a professor. And, so I knew that I liked to teach. And, I knew that I wanted to do research. And so, you know, throughout my PhD studies I had a clear goal in mind which was to return as a faculty member. There was never any doubt that that's what I wanted to do.*

Mitchell Bentley's pursuit of a PhD and his identification of a research topic emerged from his attendance at night school. He reflected:

*It was not until I started working, made the decision to go back to get a Master's degree through night school that I really renewed an interest and a passion for engineering education. And found myself drawn more and more toward the idea of finding a topic I was so passionate about that I could study it for three or four years through a PhD program.*

## Industry respondents

Similar to academia respondents, industry respondents identified their motivations for earning a PhD in engineering as fascination with something associated with their technical subject, but not research; being influenced by mentors, teachers, and/or professors; and commitment to research. Unlike academia respondents, however, industry respondents identified being influenced by a family member as an influence in their decisions to pursue a PhD.

## Fascination with their technical subject or topic

Two industry professionals, Ronald Perkins and Benjamin Kinder, acknowledged how their experiences and a desire to apply knowledge fueled their PhD pursuits. Perkins, a professional training director working in the aerospace and defense field and with a PhD in industrial engineering, noted his love of teaching at the collegiate level and the influence of his Master's experience, in which he engaged in Six Sigma experiences with "black belts" who fueled his interest in teaching.

Real-world experiences also motivated Kinder, a scientist working with a household and personal products company and with a PhD in mechanical engineering. When asked about his motivation to earn a PhD, he said that he wanted to "work on a problem that actually makes sense in a real world as opposed to work (sic) on a problem that's . . . academic in nature."

## Being influenced by mentors, teachers, and/or professors

For industry professionals, university influences, family, and friends served as positive influences in their decisions to pursue PhDs in engineering.

### Research advisors

From a university perspective, research advisors overwhelmingly influenced industry only participants to pursue advanced degrees. For Benjamin Kinder, influences included his Master's advisor and a teaching committee. Nadine Vinson, a chemical engineer and Engineer Associate working in the petroleum refining industry, noted the influence of her thesis advisor and the director of her university's engineering minority student center in her decision to earn a PhD. They encouraged her to draw upon her network, and they constantly reminded her that she had the capability to do chemical engineering graduate work.

Ginnefer Rankin, a scientist who earned a PhD in biomedical engineering, obtained her Master's degree and worked four months in industry in a manufacturing environment, which she "pretty much hated," prior to returning to graduate school. She then reconnected with her research advisor, with whom she had enjoyed doing research:

> So I was talking to her about how much I disliked the position that I had in industry. And so we started talking about me coming back and continuing the research that I was doing in her lab. And so I decided to leave the company I was working for and return to grad school to continue my research. And, which ultimately, of course, led to me getting the PhD degree.

### *Family and friends*

Family and friends also played a role in several interviewees' decisions to pursue PhDs. Bradley Simmons, a chemical engineer and Director for Process Engineering with more than 20 years of experience, shared a story about his parents and their influences as STEM professionals with advanced degrees:

> *Probably, more importantly, graduate education, be it M.D, PhD, whatever, was almost an expectation coming out of my family. I mean, my father was a PhD, even my mother who got a Bachelor's degree actually in the (19)40s, was a graduate student that pursued a Master's and as she said, 'Had I not met your father and gotten married I would have continued on for a PhD myself.' So I thought it was kind of something that I was exposed to, and were taught at least from their perspective the value of the advanced education from a pretty early age.*

Arlene Petit, a systems design engineer with less than five years of experience, eventually chose to pursue a mechanical engineering PhD during her Master's program so she would have an opportunity to enter academia or industry. Although her decision process was a long one that included her talking to "a lot of people," she referred to a friend as the major factor in her engineering PhD pursuit.

## Commitment to research

Both Nicholas Poole and Benjamin Kinder noted their affinities for undergraduate research and how those experiences motivated them to explore research topics in electrical engineering and mechanical engineering, respectively. Poole stated:

> *At the time (of undergraduate research) I was going to the (University 1) which although it's a great university it's somewhat limited in the course offerings it has because it has a fairly small electrical engineering department ... I wanted to do more related to digital signal processing and digital system design. So, I decided that the only way to do that was going to go to grad school. And since I had been doing undergraduate research I thought, you know I could be a professor. Why not? I like to hear myself talk and it would be a good way to make a living I thought. So, that was the reason why I applied to larger universities and their PhD programs that I wound up at (University 2).*

Although Poole initially thought of pursuing a career as an academic, he ultimately ended up as an industry professional after earning his doctorate.

Kinder, who obtained his undergraduate degree outside of the United States, decided to earn his PhD after he reflected on his love of studying problems in-depth. He reflected, "When I got my Bachelor's back home in India I had a career of choice- obviously go into industry to work or to get a higher degree. I'm a mechanical engineer, so I really ... enjoyed being at school." Given his research interests, he then enrolled in a Master's program.

## Academia to industry and industry to academia respondents

The thirteen respondents who had worked in both academia and industry (i.e., academia first and then industry and industry first and then academia) identified their motivations to be personal interests, being passionate about something associated with their technical subject or topic of interest; being influenced by mentors, teachers, and/or professors, experiencing prior success in graduate school, having goals that necessitated a PhD, and being passionate about research. Respondents who worked in industry first were more likely to elaborate about their motivations than respondents who worked in academia first.

### Personal interests

Respondents expressed personal interests in pursuing a PhD at some point in their educational careers. While the majority spoke specifically about their interests, some referred to them more generally. During his senior year as an undergraduate, Roland Bankston, a chemical engineering Full Professor, mentioned a desire to be challenged intellectually. Aaron Whitehurst, a Distinguished Full Professor of electrical and computer engineering at a research university, reflected on his undergraduate experience, his academic success, and his interest in pursuing more education. When given a choice between studying physics or engineering, as early as high school he chose engineering since the classes were more "organized" than his physics classes. For this reason, he noted that it was an "obvious choice" for him to pursue a PhD. Meanwhile, Eric Dillard, an Associate Professor of Materials Engineering at a research university, noted that pursuing a PhD in engineering was something he "sort of intended to do."

Although he didn't elaborate on the origin of his interest, it was apparent that he gravitated to the engineering profession and sustained interest in the pursuit of an advanced degree in materials engineering. Similarly, electrical and computer engineering Assistant Professor, Shirley Thorne, simply referred to her motivation of pursuing a PhD as a "personal goal."

Others elaborated about their reasons for pursuing PhDs. Randall Rice, a chemical engineering postdoctoral researcher working at a Master's College and University, highlighted his love of problem solving, particularly puzzles: "I love fooling around with different things, playing around with different aspects of different problems and trying to see if I can optimize it and make it better. And so the engineering side of me came out." Chemical engineering Department Chair, Mark Winkler, connected his passion for chemical engineering to his interest in medical devices. His inquisitive nature helped him to make connections between two engineering disciplines:

> For me, the first goal was that I was working in chemical engineering and I saw an area that I wanted to contribute in. And I knew that I really was interested in medical devices. And I saw it when I was working as a chemical engineer a little and I saw people working on those devices and I thought to myself, that's what I want to do- is to work on those devices. And how do I get there?

Reuben Moffit, a chemical engineering lecturer working at a research university, reiterated *why* pursuing a doctorate in engineering was most likely to relate to one's personal interest by referring to the loss of income that someone with an undergraduate engineering degree experiences by pursuing an advanced degree:

> It takes another four to six years or whatever to get the advanced degree. And, in general, all the money that you're giving up while you are in school, you are not going to get - it's not economic if you go and work out how much money you've given up these pretty modest increase in salary that you're going to get to having a Master's degree or a PhD in engineering. You know, you don't do it for economics. I'm pretty fortunate that I did it. It's something that I wanted to do. I got it. I would never be here teaching if I didn't have that PhD ... It has to be a personal intrinsic desire. It is not an economical decision.

## Being passionate about something associated with their technical subject or topic of interest

Aaron Whitehurst, Mark Winkler, Randall Rice, and academia to industry respondent, Ryan Ziegler, displayed great passions for engineering.

Whitehurst's natural affinity for engineering propelled his love of the field and its challenge motivated him to pursue an engineering PhD, becoming a successful electrical and computer engineering professor. Rice found his "calling" during his Master's program, where he worked with fuel cell membranes. Through his work with a professor during his graduate study, Winkler made interdisciplinary connections between his chemical engineering work and other aspects of engineering: "I saw that some of the skillsets that I had developed from chemical engineering, as well as just being around a lot of signal processing- more from dealing with really high fidelity-type stuff in sound and ended up being beneficial for me to make the jump from the materials and mechanics to the instrumentation side." Although he started in one area, his emergent knowledge of another area deepened his interest in pursuing a PhD. Engineering technical steward and mechanical engineer, Ryan Ziegler, connected his love of coding and teaching as the foundation for his interest in the PhD. An opportunity to be a teaching assistant grounded his interest exploring engineering graduate studies:

> My freshman year I was in the honors program, and there was one class in the honors program, it was an independent study Fortran class. And the professor who ran that class would hire former students to be TAs. So, my freshman year I took that, it was a series of three one-hour courses; I took all of them. And I was very interested in the programming and very interested in helping out other students and so I volunteered to be a TA my sophomore year and I was accepted. And then the second semester sophomore year, the person who was the lead TA, who was the grader, ended up having a conflict in his schedule with the course time, and the professor was then left finding a new grader and he asked me to do it. And so second semester sophomore year I was the grader for this series of classes. And progressively I took over essentially running the class for the professor. And I was so interested in that I decided I wanted to teach, and I wanted to teach at the university level. And, the union card for that is a PhD. And so that was my primary motivation to get a PhD.

## Being influenced by mentors, teachers, and/or professors

Most respondents who described the influence of others in their pursuit of the PhD were referring to professors or academic advisors. Philip Hays, an electrical engineering professor at a research university who focused initially on his project and scientific field as a Master's student, reflected on his growing interest and intrigue regarding the PhD and his changed career trajectory based on a professor's research guidance:

*Well, originally when I started to study at graduate school I was just interested in learning more about electrical engineering and studying for a Master's degree. But the professor I worked with ... had me working on a project related to a micro slow sensor, and I just found it extremely interesting and challenging. And he suggested that I study at (Location) and that was very attractive. So it was just originally when I started the program I was not thinking about getting a doctorate degree. I just wanted to go to industry and earn some money.*

Peter Calloway, a Chief Technology Offer working in the renewable engineering technology sector and with a PhD in electrical engineering, also made the decision to pursue his doctorate during his Master's program: "I think it was my advisor (who) encouraged (me) to pursue it, and ... at the time I was doing well in graduate school ... it seemed like if I was ever going to do it now was the best time right at the end of my Master's degree, so I thought there was no harm in trying."

Similarly, Mark Winkler started to work with a professor whose expertise was in instrumentation more so that materials and mechanics, an area in which he worked at the time. He applied his chemical engineering skillset and his newfound exposure to signal processing and high-fidelity sound to a new area of work, thereby engaging in research that would be the foundation for his post-PhD career.

Unlike previous respondents, Shirley Thorne mentioned a menagerie of personal and professional influencers at every phase of her career. She explained: "I was greatly influenced by my mother and father, in particular, my father who had a PhD in computer science and was a faculty member in that area. So along with his mentoring, and mentoring from high school teachers, and college professors, and of course colleagues, I decided to pursue a PhD in engineering."

## Experiencing prior success in graduate school

Some respondents' decisions to pursue a PhD in engineering related closely to their positive experiences in graduate school. Mark Winkler shared that although he had planned to go back to work at a pharmaceutical company, having fifteen extra credits in his Master's program encouraged him to pursue a doctorate. Reuben Moffit's success began with funding for his doctoral studies and continued as he accomplished each graduate milestone:

*I did not plan on getting a PhD. But the fact that one, I had funding, a fellowship or whatever to go to school, it was paid for, and that I was enjoying the research that I was doing in chemical engineering at (University) - and then I took the qualifying exam and passed it the first time, so I decided to continue on.*

## Having goals that necessitated a PhD

Respondents thought that obtaining a PhD would help them to obtain tangible and intangible goals. Terry Sherwood, a founder of a science consulting service and a senior lecturer at a research university with a background in chemical engineering, sought to work in an environment where he could do "something different and hopefully valuable." Mark Winkler recognized the professional and intellectual freedom that came with an engineering PhD:

*For me, it was more I felt I had to do it to get to work on the things that I wanted to get to. But it wasn't really on my radar going to grad school until I realized that that was the only way I was gonna' get to where I wanted to get to.*

Similarly, Ryan Ziegler associated the PhD with increased access such that "having a PhD will enable, (and) that not having a PhD will not enable." Shirley Thorne, however, earned her PhD with a specific long-term career objective in mind: to become an academic administrator. As such, she "felt that the degree would be necessary and vital in pursuing that career."

## Being passionate about research

Since the PhD is a research degree, it was natural for respondents to high-light their love of their research areas as reasons to pursue an engineering PhD. While Virgil Sharma, a director with a PhD in electrical engineering, found research "intriguing," Sherwood reflected:

*I was the first person in my family to go to college and so when I went I didn't really know anything about engineering but I found that I really liked it and I wanted to be able to do research. But I wasn't particularly interested in teaching. But I thought a PhD would be valuable for me to do the kind of work I wanted to do.*

Mark Winkler relished chemical engineering and honed in on an interest in medical devices. His primary question after discovering this love of research was, "How do I get there?"

## So what?

Many people interested in pursuing a PhD in engineering may not know the path required to earn that degree. The road to earning a PhD often starts with influence from someone who is aware of the doctoral pathway. Frequently, it also starts with a positive educational aspect during one's K-12, undergraduate, or Master's level education. This often occurs when a person of influence sees potential in a student and provides encouragement, funding, or some insight that presents engineering as a plausible career for that student. Unmasking the mystical aspects of the PhD and explicitly telling a student that the PhD is an option presents the degree as a possibility, often to people who have never considered pursuing advanced study in engineering. This is one reason that undergraduate research experiences, one-on-one mentoring with experienced faculty, and summer bridge programs are instrumental in allowing students to develop engineering-related professional visions. When students can see themselves as an engineer, a PhD holder, or a professor, they identify the aspects of engineering they enjoy most and often ask questions about what it takes to pursue a PhD in engineering. Such is the case of people who enjoy classroom learning and ultimately want to teach engineering.

Both research-related and non-research related passions can inform one's decision to earn an engineering PhD. Research-focused interest in the field may include curiosity about an engineering area or wanting to make connections across engineering topics that at first glance seem unrelated. The potential to advance the field of engineering resonates with many. Although the PhD is a research degree, love of something outside of research or of other intangible aspects of this degree often motivates one's pursuit of a PhD. This may include wanting to help students or society or to be a mentor and role model because of one's positive or negative college experiences. The potential to make differences in the lives of others, in the engineering profession, or in broader society, increases the likelihood that underrepresented groups will pursue an engineering PhD despite often being one of the few or only engineers in an environment.

Motivation alone is not enough to guarantee one's success and satisfaction in the pursuit of an engineering PhD. Since many undergraduate engineering degree holders can earn almost six-figure salaries after earning a bachelor's degree, the additional time required to earn a PhD − along with a potential loss of income as a graduate student during the pursuit of the degree — can be unappealing. Other limitations may include varying levels of necessity to earn a PhD, given the engineering discipline one chooses or communal respect for an engineering PhD across engineering disciplines (e.g., earning a professional engineering certification in civil engineering versus a PhD and/or MD in biomedical engineering). For this reason, early in their engineering careers students need to become aware of the requirements and negative and positive consequences of earning an engineering PhD in their engineering disciplines of choice.

## Students

- Use office hours to talk to an engineering PhD holders about their paths to success. Ask about the positive aspects of the experience as well as the negative, realizing that everyone's experience is unique.
- Ask engineering professors in your discipline what they do on a daily basis with their engineering PhDs. What percentage of time do they spend conducting research, teaching, and serving others? What advice do they have for you?
- Engage in at least one research experience as an undergraduate student. Ask a professor whose course you enjoyed if they are accepting under-graduate student researchers or is aware of multi-week research programs at other institutions. You can earn variable course credits or get paid to conduct research.

## Professionals

- Share what you do with people who may not have been exposed to engineering or to the engineering PhD is a possibility. This can occur in research seminars, one-on-one or small group meetings, webinars, or social media. Your familiarity with an engineering PhD doesn't guarantee that others are familiar with the engineering PhD. Sharing is caring.
- Identify two to three people who have the potential to earn PhDs in engineering. Take them to coffee or lunch and ask them if they had ever considered obtaining a PhD. Share the positive and negative aspects of your engineering PhD story, be available to answer questions about engineering pathways, and direct them to people and to resources that inform them about the engineering PhD process.

# References

London, J. S., Cox, M. F., Ahn, B., Branch, S. E., Torres-Ayala, A., Zephirin, T., & Zhu, J. (2014). Motivations for pursuing an engineering PhD and perceptions of its added value: A U.S.-based study. *International Journal of Doctoral Studies*, *9*, 205–227. Retrieved from http://ijds.org/Volume9/IJDSv9p205-227London0628.pdf.

# CHAPTER TWO

# The Added Value

*Since I wanted to be a faculty member I had to get a PhD. But beyond that, the PhD if it's well structured, allows you to spend a few years thinking through a very specific problem in a level that it allows you to not only become the expert in that specific problem but also gain a lot of experience as to how to think about problems, how to structure possible solutions for them- how to communicate your questions and your results in a way that will bring value to the field that you're working on...the analytical skills that are developed, the patience and just the fact that your ability to spend a lot of time on a specific problem 'til you get it just right... those experiences I think are very valuable regardless of whether or not you end up... in a career that is directly tied to what you've studied...it's more of the skill sets that you gain. So, I would say it's very valuable, but it depends on what you want to do with your life and your career.*

**Juan Cooke, PhD, Vice President of Higher Education Policy**

This chapter explores *why* someone should obtain a PhD in engineering, especially since unlike many disciplines, an engineering Bachelor's degree is terminal and allows graduates to earn above average salaries (NAE, 2004). In the vignette above, Juan Cooke reported that the added value for his earning an engineering PhD involved becoming an expert and honing his problem-solving skills. Other interviewees reflected on why they earned the PhD by answering the following question: "Based on your experience, is there any added value of getting a PhD in engineering as opposed to only a Bachelor's or Master's degree?" This *added value* is defined as opportunities, knowledge, skills, and attributes that the qualification of earning a PhD in engineering brings. Although this question focused initially on the positive aspects, or value, of earning an engineering PhD, negative aspects of getting a PhD (e.g., being overqualified to do fundamental engineering work) and neutral aspects (i.e., no added value) also emerged (London et al., 2014).

*Demystifying the Engineering PhD.*
DOI: https://doi.org/10.1016/B978-0-12-801593-3.00002-5

Positive responses about the added value of the engineering PhD involved the technical aspects of engineering, the development of professional skills, and career development and subsequent satisfaction. Technical work is defined as the ability to do scientific work or research, including the depth and the rigor of this work. Technical work also refers to additional skills engineering PhD holders need to do scientific work. Professional skills include nontechnical skills, while career satisfaction explores bigger picture aspects of earning a PhD, such as career benefits, professional development opportunities, and long-term satisfaction gained by earning a PhD. Examples of this satisfaction include access to leadership experiences (e.g., becoming a dean or leading a research team or technical lab) and exposure to new ventures or people (e.g., travel or engaging with new groups). Defining aspects of technical work, professional skills, and career satisfaction are found below:

*Scope of Technical Work*
- Becoming an expert in your field
- Understanding fundamental concepts in-depth
- Cultivating analytical thinking skills
- Developing technical writing skills
- Establishing an identity as an engineer
- Pursuing funding to execute ideas
- Being intellectually fulfilled(e.g., being a geek at heart and enjoying what you do)
- Demonstrating the ability to solve problems

*Scope of Professional Skills*
- Building confidence (e.g., inspired to continue creating and executing new ideas throughout one's career)
- Developing skills for lifelong learning
- Promoting unique ways of thinking
- Learning about yourself (e.g., organizational style, ways of thinking, etc.)
- Improving communication
- Fostering resilience
- Becoming a quick learner

*Scope of Career Development and Satisfaction*
- Impacting young scholars
- Accessing leadership opportunities during your career (e.g., becoming a dean, leading a research team or technical lab)

- Accessing additional opportunities (e.g., travel, engaging with other types of professionals)
- Added value depends on career goal
- Establishing credibility (i.e., being recognized as a content expert)
- Fiscal benefits (e.g., higher salary)
- Flexibility in designing your career (e.g., to make a transition across contexts: industry or academia; enables you to move quickly through technical roles to business roles)
- Higher starting rank
- Preparing for a faculty position (e.g., learned how to teach others, conduct research)
- Prestige
- Requirement for a profession (e.g., academic profession)

Although some academia and industry respondents professed that there was no added value of the engineering PhD, the majority of respondents lauded the benefits of this degree. Reasons cited for the PhD not being an ideal option for all engineers included not making significantly more money with a PhD, not needing a PhD to do certain types of engineering work, and not garnering professional respect from those without PhDs. Regarding the added value, only three benefits were mentioned by respondents working in more than one sector. Both academia and industry respondents noted that the added value of the engineering PhD is the ability to do scientific work. Industry and academia to industry respondents highlighted that the PhD offered access to more opportunities. Finally, academia to industry respondents and industry to academia respondents revealed that earning a PhD was a requirement for their profession. Remaining benefits of the PhD are presented throughout the rest of this chapter.

## Academia respondents

The top two reasons the PhD added value for academics included the PhD being a requirement to enter the academic profession and the PhD giving engineers opportunities to do scientific work. This correlated closely with teaching and conducting research as faculty. Entering the academic profession served as both a motivation (Chapter 1) and as an added value for earning an engineering PhD. Some academics also cited monetary and disciplinary imitations of the engineering PhD.

## Little to no added value

Academia respondents identified limitations of the PhD from monetary and career perspectives. Some thought that being wealthy was not synonymous with having a PhD. Moreover, multiple respondents agreed that getting a PhD may not be an advantageous career move for every engineer, especially given their job responsibilities and their engineering disciplines. Sherrie Roberts compared having a PhD as an electrical engineer versus a biomedical engineer by saying, "In electrical engineering I don't think there's a large added value for the PhD if you're going into industry. Now, I've talked to some colleagues of mine in biomedical engineering who don't feel that way. They feel that even in industry there's a huge added value for a PhD. I didn't see that in EE (electrical engineering)." She continued, "I don't think that having the PhD is necessarily essential to what we – what I am doing. It's required by my school, but I would say having the title "PhD" doesn't differentiate what my responsibilities would be versus anybody else's."

Surprisingly, PhD holders who did not work in industry had strong views about the benefit of the PhD for engineers working in those environments. Mark Heard acknowledged the reluctance of some companies to hire PhDs because of their higher salaries compared to other engineers. Similarly, Christopher Roe commented. I don't perceive the PhD as a way to making a lot more money unless you are one of the very few who develop a new company or a new technology and become rich out of that.

Adam Greene expressed that managers may not require the expertise of engineering PhD holders, while Samantha Ayers noted, "If you just want to go out into industry and work, I think probably the Master's is what I've seen...maybe the best value degree. That's kind of what I've been counseling my students." Finally, Roberts remarked:

> If you're thinking about going into industry I don't see a huge added value to getting the PhD. I suppose it depends on what you want to do. There are some, I suppose, very niche areas in industrial research where they would - that you might want to do that would require a PhD.

## Requirement for the academic profession

Academia respondents repeatedly confirmed the need to earn a PhD for employment in higher education environments. Although Heard explained that PhDs are needed to conduct university research, Sheryl Chambers, Samantha Ayers, and Christopher Roe mentioned their love of teaching and their earning a PhD to fulfill that love of teaching at a university level. Linda Stephens, Miranda Chilton, Stephanie Stahl, and Darnell Baker referred generally to the necessity of earning a PhD to become a professor. Stahl, an Associate Professor of Chemical Engineering working at a research university, saw an academic path as an impossible option without a PhD such that "there is no way you can become a professor," while Linda Stephens said "you cannot reach that kind of position without the PhD." Baker, an Assistant Professor in mechanical and aerospace engineering working at a research university, revealed his bias for engineering PhD holders to work in academia by professing that "it hurts you in the long run if you do a PhD and you're not academically employed."

## Ability to do scientific work

Academia respondents noted the benefit of earning a PhD to engage in research. They presented general thoughts about research, the training that emerges as a PhD holder, comparisons among Bachelor's, Master's, and PhD experiences with academic research, details about the kinds of research activities in which an engineering PhD holder engages, and the career benefits of research.

Mark Heard and Craig Daniels offered insights about PhD holders and research in general. Heard said:

> The PhD is desirable if you know you want to do research, or maybe you know you want to be part of a, let's say the direction of (a) research program. You know whether you want to be part of a research lab or a university-affiliated lab, or you may end up being in the administration and maybe ultimately your goal is to more direct and influence the direction of research rather than just do the research.

Daniels noted that "you can't do what I do without a PhD. If you want to be serious about doing research - I'm a researcher, I'm a scientist... So, to do science you have to have a PhD in my field."

Kevin Magee, Adam Greene, and Mitchell Bentley mentioned the depth of training required of engineering PhD holders. Magee reflected that "the depth of work as a PhD is so much more than even a Master's that it would be hard to imagine doing a lot of the research that's done without a PhD." He said that "it certainly makes a big difference on the depth of research or other work that you can do." Greene echoed this, "If you wanna' be involved in basic research, and really do the research yourself, you need to have the in-depth training of a PhD." Bentley rounded out this comparison of the Master's versus PhD and the expertise that the PhD brings by recalling:

> One of the professors at (Graduate University) told me one time something that I really liked that says, you get a Master's degree because you want a better engineering job. You get a PhD in engineering because you want a very specific type of engineering job.

Other respondents spoke in detail about the nuances of research with a PhD, particularly the sophistication and independence of PhD-level research. Bill Richards, an Assistant Professor of Aeronautical Engineering at a Master's College, reminisced:

> "This is the first time where I really developed research question with myself, a research question... identifying a problem to work on and I think is invaluable whether I would've learned. Through your PhD work, to be able to work independently to identify a problem to work on. I think that's skills that I obtained and developed over the PhD years."

Sheryl Chambers and Stephanie Stahl compared undergraduate research to PhD research experiences, particularly the progression of research responsibility from undergraduate to graduate education levels. Chambers noted:

> I definitely had a lot of experience doing research projects, so that as an undergraduate maybe helped with one little piece of a project, you might run some routine experiments, but through the PhD program you get to think more about experimental design. And you get to walk into things that you're not sure if they're going to work, and you try them out, and try to navigate and troubleshoot and really think about whether the path you're going down is the right one or you need to make changes.

Stahl pointed out, "What getting a PhD really prepares you to do is to guide and direct research development science; whereas with just a Bachelor's degree you are...constrained to doing something that other people conceived." In addition to PhD holders conceiving and directing projects, she articulated:

*And it [the PhD] also gives you the ability to learn to critically evaluate the liter-*
*ature so that you can really look at what other people have done and say, well*
*is it good? Is it bad? How do I use - how do I take what other people have*
*done and incorporate it into coming up with novel ideas and programs? And I*
*don't think people with a Bachelor's degree really have the education and expe-*
*rience to do those kinds of things.*

Christopher Roe and Sherrie Roberts identified the alignment of the PhD with specialized jobs in research and development in academia, industry, or government. Roberts highlighted the opportunities at government labs:

*If you're talking about doing research...in a government lab - yes, then having*
*the PhD is a big added value because it totally changes the type of work*
*that you're going to be allowed to do. You'll actually be able to do the*
*research and... there's tons of positions for Americans with PhD[s] in these*
*research labs.*

## Industry respondents

The ten industry respondents reported the most prevalent values of earning an engineering PhD as having access to more opportunities, building one's confidence, and having the ability to do scientific work or work. Industry respondents shared that earning a PhD provides mobility for engineers working in industry such that they do not have to remain in technical roles. Industry respondents also reported poor communication skills and the inability to translate theory to practice as limitations for industry professionals with engineering PhDs.

### Little to no value

Industry respondents identified PhD holders' restricted communication skills and emphases on theory more than practice as possible limitations. While Julius Kimmel, a director of research and development with a PhD in chemical engineering, professed that being a credible engineer does not mean that one can communicate with diverse audiences appropriately, Gennifer Rankin and Bradley Simmons addressed the perception that PhD holders cannot apply their expertise in industry. Regarding many PhD holders' difficulty being concise communicators, Kimmel and

Simmons expressed that PhD holders often present details of their work well, yet fail to tailor their communication to diverse audiences. Rankin alluded to engineers' personalities as reasons for communication challenges by proposing that engineering PhD holders "might be a little bit more introverted and not be really be able to express yourself as well as others." Kimmel also explained:

> I've seen some of the really great minds and great innovators who had trouble when it came to communicating. And, I think it really does take a unique skill set to be able to do that. And it just takes a lot of experience. And, I think if I can say one thing is that...it seems to be much easier for PhDs to go into great detail with sort of the deep dive presentation and communication skills. Where they seem to have more trouble is providing just succinct clear summaries of information. And, that's what I would say needs to be worked on, and needs to be a key skill. There needs to be, I would say, an excitement about what you're working on and the communication...needs to be given with enthusiasm. You need to find common ground with your audience and understand a little bit about what their motives and objectives are...try to gear your communication based on your audience.

Simmons observed that engineering PhD holders' inability to see the big picture given their emphases on depth versus breadth may impact their communication. He explained:

> One of the things that I think hampers a lot of the engineers, and actually even the PhD scientists as well, is they're so enthused about what they've got, what they've learned, that every last little detail is of equal importance to them. And, they need to learn that they need to be able to separate out those things that are of vital significance versus merely interesting. And understanding which of those elements go into that two-minute speech versus the two-hour discussion.

This inability of engineering PhD holders to communicate their work well to those outside of their technical areas aligns with the perceived lack of practicality of the PhD, as mentioned by Rankin and Simmons. Rankin divulged, "When people have a PhD, some people misperceive them as being really, really smart, but not really knowing how to move theory into something that's practical." Simmons highlighted the potential liability of the PhD, particularly when working in manufacturing, which is more applied compared to other engineering subfields:

> By having a PhD in engineering if you're working a lot around manufacturing it can actually be a liability in the fact that there's stereotypes within the com-pany that the PhDs cannot be practical thinkers. And as such have no business going anywhere near manufacturing where practicality and the ability to apply

*knowledge is a premium, and there's this misplaced perception that if you're a PhD you can't do that. . .. There are places where it can be a curse. And I know of fellow PhDs in the company who have actually hidden the fact that they had the degree until they actually established a track record in some of our manufacturing plants.*

## Access to more opportunities

Industry professionals lauded access opportunities available to them as engineering PhD holders, particularly the ability to transition within and across roles in an organization and moving between technical and non-technical roles. Nadine Vinson mentioned career advancement as a benefit of earning a PhD. She explained, "If you have the skills and the ability,... the sky is the limit. Just because you have a PhD, I don't feel you have to stay in a technical role. There are...managers and folks on the business side that just moved into a different role." Gennifer Rankin claimed that an engineering PhD offered flexibility to return to one's technical area of expertise also. She said, "Even though the work that I'm doing right now isn't exactly in the field that I studied, I could transition it back into doing biomedical research."

Both Bradley Simmons and Arlene Petit alluded to open doors that engineering PhD holders working in industry have that might not be available without the degree. Generally, Simmons realized, "At (Company), if I did not have the PhD degree there are a lot of doors... that would be closed to me." Petit noted, "It [the PhD] gives you an opportunity - whether you go into academia or into industry, there's really more opportunities."

## Building one's confidence

Stewart Oglesby, Nicholas Poole, and Benjamin Kinder lauded the confidence they gained having a PhD, particularly as they worked on project and problems that were not defined clearly. Regarding his workplace experience as a PhD holder, Oglesby, a mechanical engineer with a PhD in chemical engineering, said, "I was assigned to a project (and) it gave me the confidence that I could actually live up to the challenge, especially in the division that I found myself." Similarly, Poole, a software engineer with a PhD in electrical engineering, used a swimming metaphor such that "the research environment makes it a little bit... more comfortable just being thrown into the deep end. Just, 'Here, solve this problem.' And then you start playing with it."

Kinder mentioned the "fear factor" that is naturally part of ill-defined problems and how having a PhD reduced his fear:

> And I think... that's definitely acquired in my PhD... definitely the fear factor
> was taken out, and... when I'm looking at a new problem I look at it as an
> opportunity because I know I have the problem solving skills to go troubleshoot
> that problem or solve that problem.

He identified the differences in confidence between Bachelor's and Master's experiences with the PhD such that:

> Now I look at problems as an opportunity. And, definitely with the experience
> of doing research on a problem that nobody has solved gives you tremendous
> confidence when you try to solve very challenging problems in industry typi-
> cally...you don't get...that capability when you are in a Bachelor's degree or a
> Master's degree, and I see that with a lot of engineers here.

## Ability to do scientific work or research

Engineering PhD holders who have worked solely in industry referred to the added value of the PhD as it relates to addressing industry's research needs. Nadine Vinson said, "So that was important- being able to just do self-guided research helped the difference between that Master's and PhD. You go a little bit deeper."

Stewart Oglesby elaborated:

> If you are in research and development, then the advanced degree comes in
> very, very handy and the reason is it gives you the knowledge to be able to
> understand where everything is coming from. And then you can actually project
> and see where this is headed. And so once you go through those research and
> development work routine and you hand it over to manufacturing it becomes
> some kind of daily type of thing that you need... in R&D the advanced degree
> is a real plus.

Benjamin Kinder compared and contrasted expectations for someone with a Bachelor's degree to someone with a PhD. He explained:

> When you earn a Bachelor's degree you're solving problems but it's... laid out
> in the book... Whatever the book teaches you know, there are examples, and
> the problems in the back of the book were kind of along the same line. Seldom
> do you see problems like that in the industry. But when you earn a PhD, I think
> you're forced to acquire that skill. Because you're solving a problem that hasn't
> been solved in the past or not very many people are aware of either. You're
> really required to go out and look for information in the literature and what

*has been done, what has not been done, what's worked, what has not worked...how are you going to apply the fundamental science to solve this problem and all that stuff.*

## Academia to industry respondents

The added value of earning an engineering PhD for respondents working in academia and then transitioning to industry included having access to more opportunities than one would have with only a Bachelor's or Master's degree, becoming an expert in one's field, and having flexibility designing one's career. Opportunities and flexibility align with the potential of an engineering PhD to increase one's career satisfaction, while gaining expertise confirms the credibility of the engineering PhD.

### Access to more opportunities

Blake Greiner, Virgil Sharma, and Peter Calloway referred to the Bachelor's, Master's, and PhD when they discussed increased access as engineering PhD holders. While Sharma had no regrets earning a PhD since it opened up more opportunities for him than a Bachelor's degree, Greiner, a Principal Engineer with a PhD in mechanical engineering, recalled that at the time that he earned his PhD "the Master's was becoming more common, so a PhD would give me additional power–a type of advantage." Calloway reflected on the diversity of career options available to engineering PhD holders:

*The other value is that it opens doors to positions that you can't get without a PhD, so there are quite a few research-type positions, first of all, just academia. But secondly, the government research labs, you know, the (National Lab) and others that hire PhDs as well as you know corporate R&D labs are often looking for people with PhDs...if it's a case that you might want to do any of those positions then you must have a PhD.*

### Become an expert in one's field

Expertise is a key benefit of earning an engineering PhD. This is no surprise, however, given the purpose of the degree. To this end, Ryan Ziegler eloquently identified the differences between engineering Bachelor's, Master's, and PhD degrees:

*A Bachelor's degree- you get a very fundamental understanding of the sciences, and you can do great things with that kind of education. A Master's degree gives you a little bit more depth in an area and maybe a taste of doing research. But the PhD with the dissertation really takes things to a whole new level of having to take ownership, the idea creation, the depth to which you have to study and become an expert in that area. And having done that once it then shows that you can continue to do that throughout your career.*

Peter Calloway said that with a PhD "you gain a much higher understanding of your field... that while you get somewhat more specialized, the extra three or four years of education really gives you a firmer foundation to start your career from."

## Flexibility in designing one's career

Regarding flexibility, Blake Greiner responded, "What it [earning a PhD in engineering] does is, it lets a person move through the technical matter quicker so that they can get down to the business aspects of what they are doing."

## Industry to academia respondents

## Requirement for a profession

Numerous faculty members who transitioned from industry to academia jobs recalled the necessity of the PhD for the professoriate. Roland Bankston said, "If someone wants to become a faculty member they basically don't have a choice. So I mean it always comes up all sort of the more intellectual kind of jobs and so that's really required." Aaron Whitehurst asserted that "becoming a professor is almost entirely these days, and in the days that I started as a professor, limited to PhDs."

Shirley Thorne explained why earning a Bachelor's degree was not enough credentialing if one's career path was to become a professor, She said:

*There are also limitations if you want to be [in]academia with a Bachelor's degree. You're not necessarily going to be...eligible, but meet the preferred qualifications for an academic position in terms of teaching, in terms of research because you just haven't had that experience with a Bachelor's degree.*

Finally, both Reuben Moffit and Philip Hays mentioned the opportunity afforded with a PhD. Moffit said he is "pretty fortunate that I did it." He expounded, "It's something that I wanted to do. I got it. I would never be here teaching if I didn't have that PhD." Hays similarly acknowledges that the PhD "opened up a lot of doors." He reflected, "I couldn't get a faculty position without a PhD."

## Deeper understanding of fundamental concepts

A second theme emerging among industry to academia respondents was the benefit of an engineering PhD in obtaining a deeper understanding of fundamental concepts. Rogers believed that the PhD, unlike the Bachelor's and Master's degree, is a degree of depth. Whitt thought that the difference between the Master's and the PhD was the development of fundamentals of new concepts and the mastery of those fundamentals, respectively.

## So what?

Although there is an added value in earning a PhD in engineering, there are also unexpected limitations. First, earning a PhD does not automatically equate to extreme wealth unless someone invents a novel technology or revolutionizes an industry. Second, since a Bachelor's degree in engineering is often a terminal degree for the majority of engineering graduates and can still guarantee career success, it may be more appropriate for many engineers to earn only a Bachelor's of a Master's degree. Third, engineering PhD holders are often known best for their technical prowess, not their professional skills. As such, they may demonstrate an inability to communicate succinctly or to lead others immediately after earning their degrees, especially if no training is offered to them during their graduate programs. Regarding leadership, PhD holders do not garner respect solely because they possess a PhD, especially by those who may perceive the PhD to be a theoretical, not a practical degree.

Both academic and industry respondents mentioned that the PhD may not be a necessity for engineers working in industry. Although academic respondents spoke generally about possible mismatches between PhD expertise and industry work, industry respondents offered specific reasons that PhD holders may not fare well as industry employees. While PhD holders bring technical depth to industry, they may not know how to translate their knowledge to all audiences. There also seemed to be a perception among some non-PhD holders in industry that PhD holders cannot apply their knowledge. As such, some PhD graduates may not disclose that they have a terminal engineering degree so they can "fit" into their work environments and can be perceived as valuable members of their work teams.

Within academia, the most obvious reason engineering PhD holders reported needing a PhD was to become a university professor, primarily to teach or to conduct research. Given the credibility that the PhD brings in the academy, earning it is not optional for most engineers wanting enter the professoriate. Although many academia respondents noted their motivations for getting a PhD to be teaching, they highlighted the ability to conduct research and to influence or direct research studies and research agendas as benefit. Such research independence proved beneficial in both academic and industry settings.

Although some engineering PhD holders working in industry saw no added value of the PhD, many noted that the degree allowed easier transitions between technical and nontechnical jobs as well as opportunities to pursue more opportunities in industry. Another benefit of the PhD includes its depth, particularly its ability to position a PhD holder as an expert in an engineering area. Although the Bachelor's degree introduces students to engineering and possibly to engineering research, the Master's degree presents an initial opportunity to examine an engineering topic in-depth. The PhD, compared to the Bachelor's or the Master's degrees, offers a deeper understanding of fundamental engineering concepts. With this depth comes a PhD holder's ability to conduct original research with enhanced problem solving skills and confidence. Such expertise provides a foundation for a successful, intriguing career after earning one's PhD.

## Students

- Identify opportunities to gain breadth and depth in your pursuit of an engineering degree. Breadth may include leading projects, taking a public speaking class, or engaging with people in non-engineering disciplines.
- Engage in teaching professional development opportunities if you are interested in becoming a professor. This might involve becoming a

teaching assistant or learning about effective teaching practices through on-line modules or courses.

- Map your engineering career at Bachelor's, Master's, and PhD levels to prepare for your postgraduate career. Identify the skills and resources you need to be successful at each educational level.

## Professionals

- Share ways that you gained confidence during your PhD journey. Ask emerging scholars what their areas of concern are about earning a PhD, and offer resources that address these areas. Check in with them periodically to offer constructive feedback about their thinking.
- Present guidance to potential PhD holders about career opportunities that are available to them in industry and in academia. Connect potential mentors and mentees to improve retention in graduate education, particularly of underrepresented groups.
- Realize that a PhD is needed for advancement requires insight and foresight. Help future PhD holders think about their career goals and trajectories as early as elementary school in an effort to engage in their engineering career path.

## References

London, J. S., Cox, M. F., Ahn, B., Branch, S. E., Torres-Ayala, A., Zephirin, T., & Zhu, J. (2014). Motivations for pursuing an engineering PhD and perceptions of its added value: A U.S.-based study. *International Journal of Doctoral Studies*, *9*, 205–227. Retrieved from http://ijds.org/Volume9/IJDSv9p205-227London0628.pdf.

National Academy of Engineering. 2004. *The Engineer of 2020: Visions of Engineering in the New Century*. Washington, DC: The National Academies Press. https://doi.org/10.17226/10999.

PART II

# What Does It Mean to Be an Engineering Steward?

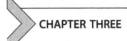

# CHAPTER THREE

# Generation, conservation, and transformation defined

## Stewardship

A primary motivation for this book is the work of Golde and Walker (2006) in *Envisioning the Future of Doctoral Education: Preparing Stewards of the Discipline*. In a series of essays, Golde and Walker invited authors to define what it meant to be a steward of six disciplines: mathematics, chemistry, neuroscience, education, history, and English. In exploring the purpose of doctoral education, they noted that a disciplinary steward is a keeper of a discipline such that they are a "scholar first and foremost in the fullest sense of the term- someone who will creatively generate new knowledge, critically conserve valuable and useful ideas, and responsibility transform those understanding through writing, teaching and application (p. 5)." Contributors were asked to answer three questions about stewardship (p. 9):

1. What constitutes knowledge and understanding in the discipline?
2. What is the nature of stewardship of the discipline?
3. How ought PhDs be educated and prepared?

Stewardship was framed in the context of three tenets, generation, conservation, and transformation. Stewardship's focus is on knowledge in the field. Generation emphasizes the creation and/or newness of knowledge in a discipline using known standards of quality and rigor. Conservation involves the preservation of knowledge and acknowledgment of the placement of one's work in the larger context of the field. Transformation communicates this knowledge to a wide variety of audiences, both in writing and orally.

This chapter extends the work of Golde and Walker by engaging respondents in questions that define stewardship in the context of engineering within academic and industry settings. Interview questions were tailored to engineering, resulting in an in-depth exploration of each stewardship tenet and include the following:

*Demystifying the Engineering PhD.*
DOI: https://doi.org/10.1016/B978-0-12-801593-3.00003-7

- Give an example of when you have created new and unique knowledge in your field. (Generation)
- What are some of the knowledge, skills, norms, attributes, ideas, questions, or perspectives an engineering PhD should understand to conduct research that meets accepted standards of rigor and quality in the field of engineering? (Generation)
- How do you apply knowledge in your field to serve others? (Conservation)
- What are the knowledge, skills, norms, attributes, ideas, questions, or perspectives engineering PhDs need to communicate with a variety of audiences? (Transformation)

# Generation

*It's very important to, and very critical that the person be able to use, display, sound rational reasoning skills so that the research that's being conducted is sound and supportable ... The reasoning that supports the conclusions have to be sound and not wishy-washy. Depending on the research, I guess the notion of properly conducted studies, and by that I mean the understanding of sound experimental design and sound experimental results, interpretation skills ... have to be there as well.*

**Gino Braxton, PhD, Senior Manager**

Gino Braxton presented core thoughts about research in engineering. He used words such as "reasoning," "experimental design," "experimental results," and "interpretation" to explain his views of engineering PhD work and to emphasize the importance of following process and using procedures that represent known research standards.

One of the goals of this book is to operationalize generation within the context of engineering. Using Golde and Walker's definition (2006, p. 10), generation refers to the abilities, skills, or acts of performing "research and scholarship that make a unique contribution and meet the standards of credible work." Since the PhD is a research degree, I expected that many responses would refer to the nuances of conducting doctoral level research in engineering. Engineering PhD respondents embodied generation by asking interesting and important questions; formulating appropriate strategies for investigating these questions; conducting investigations with a high degree of competence; and analyzing and evaluating the results of their research investigations. They also understood generation as the process of presenting and communicating their research results to others to advance the field, which is closely aligned with the stewardship tenet of transformation. Although many respondents spoke of research within their interviews, generation did not include comments in which respondents mentioned research in passing (e.g., "I teach and conduct research.") or simply referred to research as a verb (e.g., "I research chemical properties."). Examples of generation as found in analyzes included conducting detail-oriented research; possessing the insight to interpret results correctly; having the ability to conduct research or to expand upon existing research; and asking the right research questions.

Members of our research team explored stewardship in the development of a strategic blueprint for engineering graduate students (Berdanier et al., 2016). As such, Fig. 3.1 displays all mentions of generation within

| Stewardship Tenet: Generation Producing new knowledge that contributes to the field | | |
|---|---|---|
| Themes | Components | Definitions |
| Research (any element of the research process: not necessarily novel contributions) | Improve on prior knowledge or processes | Improving products or processes (often in service of solving a problem), filling in gaps in competency or skill, and working to exceed the performance or efficiency of existing materials |
| | Employ rigorous research methods | Knowledge of scientific method, designing appropriate experiments to test well-developed hypotheses |
| | Problem analysis | Assessing a problem and analyzing potential solutions; fully understanding a problem through direct experience |
| | Data analysis | Knowing how to analyze data using appropriate statistical or qualitative techniques; interpreting and drawing relevant conclusions |
| Contributions to the field (specifically unique and navel contributions) | Vision | Understanding how research fits into the broader fiels; recognizing boundaries and when boundaries can be pushed |
| | Impact | Conducting/publishing research that improves or advances knowledge or has practical impact; something that can elicit change |
| | Publications, presentations, and patents | Making viable, unique, and relevant contributions to the discipline through Intellectual Property, publication, or communication venues |
| Characteristics | Personal | Characteristics soecific to the individual (and not to job training), (e.g. detail-orientation, strong work ethic, work style) |
| | Professional | Characteristics that reflect skills unique to job training (e.g. fundamental engineering knowledge, rigorous methods skills, critical assessment) |
| | Ability to teach others to generate knowledge | Mentoring or advising undergraduate or graduate students, specifically in regard to the development of research skills |
| Knowing the field | Knowing the field | Possessing deep disciplinary knowledge and experience which allows one to ask relevant and meaningful questions |

**Figure 3.1** Generation Themes, Components, and Definitions Identified across Respondents (Berdanier et al., 2016).

interview transcripts. Although this chapter highlights questions that deliberately asked about stewardship, Chapter 4 includes instances of stewardship identified as characteristics and expectations of engineering PhD holders. As such, interview questions eliciting responses across academic and industry include the following:

• Give an example of when you have created new and unique knowledge in your field, and

• What are some of the knowledge, skills, norms, attributes, ideas, questions, or perspectives and engineering PhD holder should understand to conduct research that meets accepted standards of rigor and quality in the field of engineering?

## Academia respondents

For many respondents who worked in academia, contributions to their technical work represented much of their generation. Many general responses overlapped with the stewardship tenet of transformation. Despite the expectations for academics, George Murray was the sole academic who mentioned authoring journal papers, patenting, and contributing to intellectual property as unique contributions to the field.

Examples of impactful contributions that respondents made in their areas of research included interfacing biology with engineering to understand what makes some cells strong protein producers (Stephanie Stahl); designing materials that used negative stiffness to absorb energy (Mark Heard); using ocular biomechanics to understand glaucoma in a better way (Craig Daniels); creating a device to alleviate some of the symptomatic behavior of individuals on the autism spectrum (Mitchell Bentley); discovering a new form of protein developed for Parkinson's disease (Linda Stephens); designing normal materials to sense toxins in food and water (Linda Stephens); and modeling the impact of optical interconnection technologies on parallel processing systems (Juan Cooke). Although these topics differed, academia increased the likelihood that contributions would be made given researchers' reliance on grant funding to support their research enterprises.

A benefit of conducting research in a university setting was engineering PhD holders' engagement with students either in a research apprenticeship or in the application of engineering-related concepts to a classroom environment. Other generation contributions included interactions with students. Miranda Chilton, Stephanie Stahl, and Sherrie Roberts described how they translated research to practice for students in their courses. Chilton used knowledge she gained from a funded NSF grant to create hands-on experiences for her engineering students:

> I am not at all afraid ... to try different types of teaching so I'm not modeling the way I was taught. I try doing different things, and I reach out looking for people - 'cause I would rather not take the time to develop it, so I ... look and see if anybody else has already created something that I could use and try for other teaching methods ... I found, for example, someone that got an NSF grant that has created a series of hands-on experiences to help students learn heat transfer versus just lectures about the theory. And figuring out how to roll that into a traditional classroom 'cause I don't really have a lab space to use. So that's fun to do.

Stahl explained how involving her student in novel research that had the potential to result in patents:

> I actually sent a student to work at a company in England. And she did really beautiful work so I think there really is a lot of ... scientific discovery. We had done some things that have been more invention. We filed a couple of patent

*disclosures on a collaborative project that I had with a company. We didn't actually get patents for a variety of reasons. But we did actually come up with some real, some novel technologies.*

Roberts spoke of her cross-institutional curricular innovation:

*I do a lot of work on these courses developing a lot of new things; developing new labs. I work with ... somebody that I used to work with at (Former University) who's now also a professor at my current institution, and we are doing something totally different. For example, I teach logic labs that nobody else is doing. What I do now is more ... small-scale curricular innovation ... hasn't been done before at my school. And then some large-scale [curricular innovation that] hasn't been done anywhere.*

## Industry respondents

Many of the generation themes among industry professionals represented contributions to the field--particularly the impact of research inside and outside of an organization--along with commercializing, publishing, and patenting research innovations. Given this focus on creating knowledge that impacts others, several of the generation codes overlapped with transformation codes.

## Publishing

Stewart Oglesby and Gino Braxton, a Senior Manager with a PhD in industrial engineering, offered perspectives about publishing practices in industry. Oglesby spoke about coal combustion publications he co-authored along with practical applications of his work. In speaking about ways to stabilize glass sheets, he highlighted differences between publishing in academia and industry, particularly the role that a legal department in industry played prior to publishing:

*There's a literature review work that I did that has been published on how to surely apply the concept [of stabilizing glass sheets]. We have ... since then made several improvements. But that is still being looked at by the legal department before we can publish.*

Rather than publishing in traditional journals, Braxton presented thoughts about cooperative education students publishing their research findings:

*In my tech research days ... I was in that role for probably about 10 years, and I had generally three co-ops working for me at any time, co-op engineers, and they would be given any number of problems to go look at. And they were expected and required to create, or write-up their results, in the form of a white paper and that had very ... strict guidelines in how that structure was set. And there was a lot of knowledge generated in that world about how our business worked or how candidate solutions might actually behave in the real world.*

## Commercializing and patenting

In the same way that publishing differed across industry and academia respondents, an additional expectation of industry professionals was to commercialize and patent their innovations. Each example highlighted the diversity of engineering innovations and the impact of them within and across engineering disciplines. Julius Kimmel described the commercialization of products and the process:

*The innovation that we had developed was a way to really reduce the particle sizes of and optimize the hardness and morphology of ... these abrasive particles ... that led to the commercialization that was very successful for that generation of products.*

*Now the products have since moved on to other technologies. Things change and so these products while asked for a certain period of timemany times they go away and we have to keep changing and adapting to those sorts of market forces and market changes.*

Stewart Oglesby discussed the patenting process for an environmental project in the household and personal products company in which he worked. He explained efficiency results for his company:

*The (other) concept that I came up with in the environmental project that I was supporting, also recently we got a patent out of that. And the patent had to do with some of the material changes we had to do to improve the capture selective removal of mercury from coal combustion ... There are a whole bunch of processes out there that people use to capture mercury from fuel gas, but usually the capture efficiency is about maybe 40–50% efficiency. We came up with a process where we gave them the material that we actually put in the substrate. We could capture upwards of above 85% efficient.*

Gennifer Rankin also expounded about her patenting experience for a new material that would enhance consumer comfort:

*We actually filed a patent for a new technique that could be used to aperture, or put tiny holes, in an elastic rubber knit material to make it breathable, which would make it more comfortable for consumers to use.*

Finally, Benjamin Kinder referred to a winding method that was published and was awaiting a patent in his company. To understand what winding was and why it is an important problem to address, he explained:

> Winding is, for example, if you take ... a tissue paper roll, that's a long roll ... Just imagine the size to be about maybe three meters wide, say 120 inches wide by about 50 inches in diameter. That's the size of the rolls that we make day in and day out. And it's very important that we wind it just right, because we don't want to lose any of the material that we put on that roll. We want to use every ounce of that material because otherwise it's just a waste and it equals to dollars.

> We typically have waste associated with long roll tissues that's been going on for the last 10 years, and we were able to identify that as the source - the long roll as the source, and we were able to invent a new method to wind rolls differently that eliminated that problem ... We were able to create a first of a kind method to solve one of the most challenging problems from a winding standpoint that we've had for the last years.

## Other contributions to the field

Improved organizational processes and university-industry collaborations illustrated other examples of generation among industry only respondents. Arlene Petit spoke of internal communications as an aspect of generation:

> It's hard ... to publish on things when you're in industry. So I ... had done a lot of that, so it's ... been internal things where ... in our own laboratory here at work we've done a lot of process improvement. As a team, we've been involved in basically changing a lot of the processes internally; so that has been really where it was kind of recognized at the expert level for making the processes better at the company.

Benjamin Kinder offered a valuable perspective about university-industry relations and cross-collaborations. He described, "We involve universities too, when we do open innovation projects where we deliberately involve universities to solve certain problems where either we don't have resources to solve, or we don't have the expertise to solve."

## Knowing the field

Both Bradley Simmons and Gino Braxton shared insights about the technical expertise that industry professionals were expected to exhibit. Much about knowing the field related to processes and interpretation of information as an engineering PhD holder with foci on big picture problem solving, logic, and rationality. Simmons reflected:

*They [engineering PhD holders] need to be able to think ... multiple steps ahead. I see too many PhDs that run their research program literally an experiment at a time, and they don't think in terms of, 'Okay, when I run this experiment, one, what question am I actually trying to answer? Two, is the experiment itself properly designed to answer that question? Three, what are the possible results that I could get from this experiment? Depending on the result what direction would I go?' Which is where I get into thinking ahead a little bit as opposed to allowing the last result to dictate where you go next-- Which is kind of a shorthand way of saying that the PhDs need to have a strategy around which they're actually trying to do their discovery or plan their problem solving.*

Braxton also provided details about engineering PhD holders' expertise as it relates to generation:

*It's very important to, and very critical that the person be able to use, display, sound rational reasoning skills so that the research that's being conducted is sound and supportable ... The reasoning that supports the conclusions have to be sound and not wishy-washy. Depending on the research, I guess the notion of properly conducted studies, and by that I mean the understanding of sound experimental design and sound experimental results, interpretation skills-- I think have to be there as well.*

## Academia to industry respondents

The majority of academic to industry respondents identified patenting as their primary contributions to generation, although Blake Greiner also referred to trade secrets. With one patent and another pending, Ryan Ziegler described his patent as "an acknowledgment by the U.S. Government that I developed something new." Those patents were "ideas that came out of trying to solve problems that we were facing with certain products, and in solving those problems we came up with new solutions." Peter Calloway mentioned that his patents involved techniques to improve products, to improve the efficiency of power conversions, and to reduce product costs.

## Industry to academia respondents

Most industry to academia to industry respondents referred to their contributions to the field, which resulted in generation and conservation occurring simultaneously. Patenting was a recurrent demonstration of generation, confirming the importance of producing and sharing technical knowledge for engineering PhD respondents working in industry.

## Patents

Roland Bankston, Shirley Thorne, Mark Winkler, and Philip Hays highlighted the patents that they have received for their research contributions across both industry and academic settings and even several years after conducting the initial work. For the latter, Winkler noted that the dissertation work he conducted ten years prior to this interview was tested in patients almost a decade later and had been improved so it had recently become patentable. Thorne worked on a team at a national laboratory to file two patents on the semi-conductor process and inductor integrated processing. These inductors are used in building IC (integrated circuit) chips and building IC technology. Bankston received two patents, one for paper making and another that involved the manipulation of molecules on a surface that could control the properties of a transistor that was being manufactured. He reflected on how his technology impacted the pharmaceutical industry:

> So a lot of the technology I have developed is used, has been used and is used, on real pharmaceutical compounds to make higher quality pharmaceuticals and to make them cheaper basically; focusing more on quality and reliability ... reliability to making sure that you produce the same drug or compound or the same structure every time That's had a pretty big impact on society and humanity.

> And then the reason this works is 'cause ... I develop technology ... I do have a technology that allows people, other people, to make the processes much more efficient and produce much higher quality products much more reliably.

Hays' patent incorporated research he conducted in academia with his graduate student. He described the process from beginning to end:

> We had to design a valve for a fuel cell. And so the sponsor wanted us to make this valve as small and as low power as possible. And valves up to that point had been made with separate components that are assembled. And so with my graduate student we came up with a design where we could integrate the actuator coil and the fluid flow channels onto a single substrate. And we filed a patent on that. We first filed an invention disclosure on that. And then we built it here, built first the actuator, and then we built the actuator with the

*flow channel; demonstrated its performance. And the patent was granted. I was very happy that the patent was granted for that valve design.*

## Technical contributions

Engineering PhD holders must demonstrate technical expertise to earn their degrees. Terry Sherwood reiterated the importance of engineering PhD holders making "a genuine contribution to the field," which involved originality, hard work, and doing more than simply following instructions. Reuben Moffit and Aaron Whitehurst described their unique contributions to engineering as PhD holders. Moffit worked across two universities to develop a theoretical model at a second university with novel, experimental data collected at the first university. Whitehurst reflected holistically about his contributions across his career in an effort to influence his field:

*One thing I've done in my career is, I've figured out a methodology that builds hardware that operates in these very fast optical signals and reshapes them under computer control according to a user's specifications. In my own case, I had some of my own ideas about high-speed communications applications. And I pursued some of those. And some at least have some influence.*

## So what?

Generation in the context of engineering did not focus solely on the creation of knowledge. Academia respondents focused heavily of their unique contributions to the field being the engineering work they conducted and ways that they engaged their students in research development or apprenticeships. Industry respondents emphasized the applications of their work as generation, particularly commercializing technology, publishing, and patenting their innovations. Industry applications were not limited to business with external stakeholders but also involved streamlining of processes and university-industry collaborations. There was an expectation that engineering PhD holders in industry were technically competent and understood the process for making sound technical decisions. Respondents in all sectors referred to patenting, but engineering PhD holders with industry experiences most often mentioned patents as their unique research contributions. More than once, respondents focused on the need for engineering PhD holders to demonstrate sound, rational, concrete processes in the development of genuine contributions to the field. Given the precision of engineering and its emphasis on problem solving and analytical thinking, this is not surprising.

## Students

- See Berdanier, Tally, Branch, Ahn, and Cox (2016) for a blueprint for graduate students' development of generation.

## Faculty

- Explore the generation expectations in your current position, possibly in your promotion and tenure document. Use your generation outcomes to connect to conservation and transformation efforts.
- Ensure that students comprehend the fundamentals of a discipline rather than focusing solely on memorizing concepts and formulas. Identify ways for them to connect what they are learning with what they will be expected to do later in their careers.

## Industry professionals

- Reflect on what generation means to you and how you create unique knowledge in your field. If you are not engaging in activities that promote generation, yet you want to do so, speak with a supervisor and create short-term and long-term plans to enhance your generation.

## Conservation

*The second [characteristic] is a strong understanding of the fundamentals so that you have the building blocks, you're aware of what's been done in the past, that - the integrity piece comes into that in that you're not trying to pass off what other people have done as your own ideas, and you're really aware of where others have been and where the open spaces may be.*

**Ryan Ziegler, PhD, Engineering Technical Steward**

Although Ryan Ziegler responded to a question about the characteristics that he thought engineering PhD holders should possess to conduct research that met accepted standard of rigor and quality in the field of engineering, his response aligned closely with the stewardship definition of conservation. Golde and Walker (2006) defined conservation as exhibiting "an understanding of the history and fundamental ideas of the discipline," having "the responsibility for maintaining the continuity, stability and vitality of the field," and "understanding how their discipline can speak to important questions" (p. 10—11).

Berdanier et al. (2016) analyzed conservation codes across all transcripts and interview questions (Fig. 3.2), noting that conservation within the context of engineering links closely to one's demonstration of technical skills and technical leadership along with their knowledge of the field. Although technical skills reflect one's mastery of fundamentals and other expectations of technical prowess, technical leadership includes teaching and having the ability to assess the relevance of information created in the field. Finally, knowledge of the field relates to one's ability to link knowledge to current trends, to process and employ literature in the field, and to understand how to "do" something with that knowledge in a way that preserves its relevance in the field.

To identify what conservation looks like in engineering, respondents were asked, "How do you apply knowledge in your field to serve others?" This question was presented given conservation's role as a stabilizing force in the field and since the application of one's role in service provides opportunities for engineering professionals across a variety of sectors to describe how they engage with and preserve fundamental knowledge in the discipline. Unlike responses for generation and transformation, however, conservation responses were not expounded on greatly by engineering PhD holders.

| Stewardship Tenet: Conservation | | |
|---|---|---|
| Preservation of disciplinary knowledge and history | | |
| Themes | Components | Definitions |
| Technical skills (general) | Mathematical fundamentals | Strong understanding of statistics; mathematical modeling |
| | Engineering fundamentals | Understanding the history of the field; knowledge of foundational engineering problem solving components (e.g. engineering analysis, problem recognition, application of science, math, and engineering principles, generate engineering solutions) |
| | Expertise | Depth of knowledge; being at the forefront of discipline |
| | Scientific method | Apply scientific method, including generation of hypotheses, experimental design and execution, and data analysis |
| | Data analysis | Analyze and interpret data generated through disciplinary research |
| | Technology | Identify and use relevant instrumentation or programs to achieve research objectives |
| Technical leadership | Teaching | Build understanding or knowledge of the field in the classroom. Includes generating relevant examples, assessing level of learning |
| | Assessing relevance to the field | Guidance of discipline through gatekeeper roles (e.g. serving as an editor or journal reviewer, using knowledge to inform policy, service to the institution, creating new programs, serving on qualifying committees, or anticipating impact of policy on discipline) |
| Knowing the field | Literature | Reading, analyzing, and utilizing published literature in the field |
| | Identify current technology and trends | Identify current topics/issues and current trends in a discipline's innovation, and be able to recognize state-of-the art technologies |
| | Synthesize existing information | Integrate information from different areas/sources to solve problems |
| | Use multiple resources from diverse sources | Find and use relevant information from a variety of online, physical, or human resources |

**Figure 3.2** Conservation Themes, Components, and Definitions Identified across Respondents (Berdanier et al., 2016).

## Academia respondents

To academics, conservation connected to teaching, knowing the fundamentals of the field, and comprehending literature so one has an awareness of how they are making technical contributions in an effort to translate information to others who many not possess an engineering PhD. Teaching, a somewhat obvious illustration of conservation, occurred not only in the higher education classroom, but at the K-12 level, and even in the form of mentoring. Sheryl Chambers referred to "being able to bring an understanding or knowledge about the field to the classroom" and providing relevant examples for students to discuss along with interesting case studies for them to consider.

Catrina Benson presented her teaching contributions in the development of a robotics minor, her judging high school robotics competitions, and her desire to mentor African-American engineering PhD students.

Although she felt obligated to increase the pipeline of African-American female engineering PhDs, she identified a limitation in her demonstration of conservation to be her pre-tenure faculty rank. With a limited number of hours in a day, she admitted that although she wanted to mentor more female undergraduate or graduate students to pursue the PhD, she anticipated that those roles are in the purview of senior faculty, mainly Associate or Full Professors. She explained the current activities in which she engaged as an Assistant Professor:

> Probably one of the best things I do to apply knowledge in my field to serve others is because my PhD area was in robotics, is we have a multi-disciplinary robotics minor, and I serve as a judge for the first robotics competition, which is a high school competition where students work together to introduce them to science and engineering, and they build and program a robot to meet some specific task. So that's probably one of my primary service areas that I think is also related to my profession. I do other things for service at my school, but I don't think any of them ... necessarily require any special technical skill, just for my body to be there and to give the time.

Both Stephanie Stahl and Juan Cooke offered specific examples about ways that engineering PhD holders might conserve knowledge. Stahl referred to evaluating literature critically to examine if what others have done is "good" or "bad" and to ask, "How do I take what other people have done and incorporate it into coming up with novel ideas and programs?" Cooke emphasized the value of using high ethical standards to conduct research so doctoral dissertations are "new and valuable work that can be studied and moved on by others."

Cooke also demonstrated technical leadership by noting relevance of the field to policy:

> If I look at it from the standpoint of my knowledge of engineering education, then I would say that the way I apply my knowledge is by bringing in the experiences that I have had in engineering education, and the other areas that I have worked on the past few years — bringing that experience on the practice side of education, bringing it and letting it influence or inform the policy decisions that we are advocating for now.

> ... We're weighing in on the national debates surrounding the regulation of for-profit colleges. We're weighing in on Congress' threat of cutting program funding ... We're weighing in on states that are considering establishing performance funding models that would determine whether or not higher education could get ... additional funds based on their graduation rates, and

*retention rates, and what not. And, we're looking at policy positions and actual policy recommendations for each one of these topics that I just mentioned.*

*The experience that I have had as an educator in the engineering field ... is very useful in allowing us to craft policy recommendations and take policy positions that are grounded ... in reality — that take into account the realities of shared governance in academic settings for example, which is something that a pure policy person would not be able to do.*

## Industry respondents

Surprisingly, when industry respondents were asked about a time they applied knowledge to serve others, it did not map directly to this study's definition of conservation. Instead of focusing on preserving knowledge in the profession, many responses mapped better to transformation, particularly to the application of knowledge, skills, insights, and findings. Stewart Oglesby, however, talked about conservation beginning with hypothesis testing after researching what others have done in the field and exploring what drew them to that work.

## Academia to industry respondents

One respondent, Ryan Zeigler, contributed greatly to the operationalization of conservation in his service and as a technical steward. He discussed a unique perspective about technical leadership via his service as the new chairman of an industrial advisory council for a new engineering department in a new field at his alma mater. He saw himself as an activist who could provide an external voice to the department as an advocate, advisor, and supporter. He said that "my role will be to ... facilitate additional activities ... beyond that I think there's really a recruiting role to some extent of trying to find other people to serve on the council, to make sure that ... we broaden the voice, and that we provide the best support to the school that we can." Zeigler also noted the importance of technical skills and the integrity needed to conduct research. His advice to engineering PhD holders is that "you're not trying to pass off what other people have done as your own ideas and you're really aware of where others have been and where the open spaces may be."

## Industry to academia respondents

Foundational knowledge about one's technical area proved to be strongly connected to teaching. Teaching was enacted in multiple ways and included lifelong learning in an effort to preserve one's field. For example, Eric Dillard presented teaching as a way that he conserves the field. He also alluded to transformation such that engineering PhD holders needed to exhibit an additional awareness to adjust their teaching to an appropriate level for their students and to possess a depth of technical knowledge in doing this. He noted that when teaching, "a mistake a lot of people make ... is they don't understand the level at which they need to teach the material." Randall Rice connected teaching and learning as a professor such that:

> On the one hand I'm teaching; on the other hand I'm learning. So on the one hand I'm using the skills that I already have to help bring up and teaching those that are wanting to become researchers, and those are developing those skills as researchers. And then on the other hand, I'm learning for those who've already been in the field ... 10, 20, 30 years, and listening to what they've learned and try to apply it to what I already know.

He also acknowledged the importance of learning from more experienced instructors to refine his research skills and to expand his knowledge base. Within those exchanges with experts, when he lacked understanding, he asked, "Can you give me a sense of what am I missing? Am I missing key pieces of the puzzle here?"

For teaching, Rice said:

> So having to ... sow those seeds within them [students] early so that they can go forward and then get comfortable, actually giving them a little small research problem, design their experiments, carry out their experiments, get the results, and then take the time to sit down and analyze the results. To understand, "Does this seem valid? Does the data I have correspond or correlate well with what's been published before?"

Roland Bankston also explained how he used his technical skills in his job to increase product quality, to increase throughput, and to "de-bottle" processes and to ultimately guide others to sound technical solutions:

> So then they will call me in and then I will give them a bunch of technical problems. And the technical problems are such that I don't need to know the molecular structure of the compound to understand the problem.

*And then I'll come back and I'll say, "These are things that I would try ... that you should look into." So, "Take this measurement. If it gives you this it tells you that you should try this. If the measurement tells you this you should try this. If you try this particular technology, that maybe I didn't develop maybe somebody else developed, if you try this other technology." So I give them ... different ideas of experiments to gain information that will - or technologies that they should use to de-bottleneck their process.*

Both Rice and Winkler connected conservation and transformation by mentioning the importance of knowing fundamentals before communicating those fundamentals to others. Rice noted, "The first thing that a person needs to understand [is the fundamentals] ... If you can't do that you're not going to be able to effectively communicate your results to the broad spectrum." Describing the needs of a Bachelor's program at his university, Winkler said that an engineering PhD holder should understand what students need to know to move them in the direction they must go.

## So what?

*Conservation* was not expounded on extensively by respondents in this study. Technical expertise, or knowing the fundamentals of the field, was foundational for comprehending literature and demonstrating expertise as an engineering PhD. Teaching came up as an aspect of conservation that extended beyond typical classroom teaching such that respondents highlighted the importance of translating knowledge appropriately for students in courses, being reflective about ways to transfer years of engineering expertise into applications that students can comprehend and apply, and scaffolding knowledge so students can garner incremental successes as they learn engineering fundamentals. People working in industry offered specific examples about ways they conserved knowledge via their engaging in an advisory capacity for an engineering department and how they linked old and new knowledge by understanding the field. Conservation did not operate in isolation but involved students, partners, and mentors. Because of this, there was an element of lifelong learning so that checks and balances occurred regarding technical knowledge acquired and passed on to others. Conservation of knowledge preceded communication of this knowledge (i.e., transformation).

## Students

- See Berdanier et al. (2016) for a blueprint for graduate students' development of conservation stewardship.

## Faculty

- Determine which concepts are appropriate to introduce to students at various levels (e.g., undergraduate vs. graduate) and across contexts (e.g., classroom vs. research settings).
- Engage in lifelong learning via professional development activities. Given the nature of engineering, connect with experts outside your area of expertise to make connections between your field and other fields.

## Industry professionals

- Connect with faculty at universities to stay abreast of current courses, techniques, and advancements in your field.

## Transformation

*One of the things that I think hampers a lot of the engineers, and actually even the PhD scientists as well, is they're so enthused about what they've got, what they've learned, that every last little detail is of equal importance to them. And, they need to learn that they need to be able to separate out those things that are of vital significance versus merely interesting. And understanding which of those elements go into that two-minute speech versus the two-hour discussion.*
**Bradley Simmons, PhD, Director of Process Engineering**

Golde and Walker (2006, p. 11) define transformation as "teaching in the broadest sense of the word" which involves "representing and communicating ideas effectively and clearly . . . to a variety of audiences in oral and written form." This somewhat vague definition offered an opportunity to identify numerous examples of teaching across sectors. Fig. 3.3 (Berdanier et al., 2016) explores instances of stewardship for all interview questions, and identified five overarching themes, (1) teaching, (2) verbal communication skills, (3) written communication skills, (4) communication (general), and (5) application of knowledge across all transformation codes.

Responses from a single transformation question, "What are the knowledge, skills, norms, attributes, ideas, questions, or perspectives engineering PhDs need to communicate with a variety of audiences?," resulted in responses being classified in four ways: (1) communication, (2) multi-disciplinarity, (3) teaching, and (4) the application of knowledge, skills, findings, and insights. *Communication* involves sharing knowledge clearly with a wide variety of audiences in written and oral forms. *Multi-disciplinarity* includes awareness and understanding of other disciplines. *Teaching* is multifaceted in its transcending settings (e.g., occurring outside of the classrooms) but excludes basic teaching responsibilities (e.g., grading or holding office hours). It ultimately represents the breaking down of complex ideas and passing knowledge on about a content area regardless of context. Finally, the *application of knowledge, skills, findings, and insights* involves both direct and indirect ways that information is shared. The four aspects of transformation are explored across engineering sectors.

## Academia respondents

Academics referred to broader impacts in technical areas and in their outreach to non-engineering communities as ways that they share knowledge

| Themes | Stewardship Tenet: Transformation<br>Translating expertise to a variety of audiences | |
| | Components | Definitions |
|---|---|---|
| Teaching | Tailoring communication to audience | Recognizing audience's level of knowledge, perspective, break down complex technical problems to basic principles |
| | Non-classroom teaching | Teaching, training, or education of audiences outside a classroom setting |
| | Classroom teaching | Teaching, within a traditional engineering higher education classroom |
| | Mentoring | Formal or informal guidance of younger or less-experienced engineers |
| | Administration | Program direction and leadership related to education |
| | Outreach | Informal education with the intent to expose outside groups to engineering and/or science principles |
| Verbal communication skills (public and private) | Presentation skills | Characteristics related to public communicationin presentations: (e.g. articulateness, eye-contact, use of media, content, etc.) |
| | Conferences | Willingness to engage with disciplinary community in conference settings |
| | Concise communication | Judgment of what information is relevant and necessary |
| | Communicating appropriately for situations and audiences | Management of professional discourse among colleagues and collaborators, including method and mode of communication, roles in business or research meetings, interactions with customers |
| Written communication skills (public and private) | Journal publications | Ability to write for scholarly audience by publishing new knowledge in scholarly journals |
| | Patents | Ability to file patents in order to protecting intellectual property |
| | Concise communication | Ability to write in a succinct and clear manner |
| | Appropriate mode of communication | Understanding appropriate situations in which to use different modes of communication (e.g. face-to-face communication, phone, email, videoconference, written report) |
| | Research proposals | Ability to write research proposals to obtain research funding |
| Communication (general) | Personal attributes | Skills related to overall personal presentation during communication (e.g. voice, poise, confidence, articulateness, conciseness and non-verbal communication employed during any form of communication) |
| | Break down complex ideas | Ability to dissect ideas into most basic components |
| | Tailor communication to audience | Communicate effectively with audiences of different needs and knowledge levels (e.g. management, customers, colleagues, students, public) |
| Applicatioi knowledge | Recognize impact | Understand the impact of engineering decisions on stakeholders' interests (e.g. profitability, innovation) |
| | Commercialization | Translate research findings to business application |
| | Patents | Protect generated knowledge through patent |
| | Broader impacts | Understand impacts of technology beyond immediate benefits to stakeholders |

**Figure 3.3** Transformation Themes, Components, and Definitions Identified across Respondents (Berdanier et al., 2016).

in their field. They also emphasized the importance of communicating with people outside of current academic circles, working in multidisciplinary spaces, teaching in classrooms outside of nontraditional environments, and knowing how to translate technical information appropriately to students.

# The application of knowledge, skills, findings, and insights
## Broader impacts (technical)

Several respondents explained how their research transforms their fields. Although most people outside of engineering may not comprehend the technical nuances of this work, it is presented in the voices of respondents to highlight their passion for this work and to present how they define contribution of this work to others. George Murray summarized his transformation contributions as commercial activities, economic development, and patenting, while Linda Stephens noted that the impact of the research was physically beneficial to the society. Christopher Roe offered a big picture perspective about the potential impact of these technical projects:

> Sometimes the projects have very clear implications for society like when you're researching new ways of treating a disease. And sometimes they don't. Sometimes you're working on some things that are more abstract but potentially could lead to new discoveries.

He further described his work with nanoparticles and reasons that this work is transformative:

> Right now we are working with using … magnetic nanoparticles as probes of the mechanical properties of complex fluids. So nano scales as costly measurements. And this is rather unique compared to other techniques because it can go to very small end scales which other techniques are not suitable for. And also, it's measures the rotational movement of the particles, not the translational movement.

Craig Daniels, Stephanie Stahl, Darnell Baker, and Mitchell Bentley highlighted the applications of their research in glaucoma, recombinant protein production, environmental contamination, and assistive technologies, respectively. Daniels explained:

> I'm a biomedical researcher, so the reason I did this was to try to understand glaucoma as a disease. It's the second leading cause of blindness in the world behind cataracts. And so my work is all focused on trying to improve clinical care, which of course is a very insidious disease. It affects about four percent of the population in the United States over 65, over 60 actually. So this is a big time disease. And so my job is focused on trying to help understand that disease and thereby improve clinical care for all those people who are unfortunately affected by it.

Meanwhile, Stahl presented an overview of her work:

> The focus of my research is on recombinant protein production. I do a fair amount of collaboration with the biotech industry. So I would say that's probably the biggest service … in that sense. One of the things that happens in the biotechnology industry is that their timelines are so tight that they really don't have a lot of time to do basic process science. So that's really a significant

*contribution that I think I make ... I tell people we're doing the experiments that the people in industry would like to do but they don't have the time to do.*

Similarly, Baker summarized the impact of his research:

*My only research relates to environmental contamination ... My ultimate result is to provide clean air and clean water for everybody to breathe and drink. That's how I serve others. It readily impacts human beings and the ultimate goal is to provide better resources for everybody.*

Bentley not only spoke of his research with assistive technologies for people with special needs but illustrated how he connected this work to learning opportunities for his students:

*I think the way that I do that [serve others] is to include in my classes and my research a direct connection to the students, what they're working on now, and how it would be used at some point in time in the future by them or by humanity.*

*I do a lot of work with assistive technologies for individuals that have special needs, either through autism or physical disabilities. And so I use a lot of examples of how the engineering work that the students are doing either in the classroom or the research would directly impact individuals using assistive technologies.*

*For example ... we're adding a research project on low power where if you have something that is lower power ... the individual with the disability would be able to use it for a longer period of time without additional support or assistance.*

*I think that by tying everything we do for the students to a long-term goal that directly benefits society, benefits not only the students in their education process but it also helps society because their needs are being directly seen by the students as they do the work. It further motivates the students to perform at a higher level.*

### Broader impacts (outreach)
Outreach among academic respondents included several service learning projects, particularly Engineers without Borders (Kevin Magee and Bill Richards), outreach with local communities (Sheryl Chambers and Samantha Ayers), and outreach with K-12 students (Sherrie Roberts).

Roberts summed up her reason for doing outreach as "helping other people ... outside of engineering learn about engineering and hopefully get involved." Magee and Richards referred to Engineers without Borders when they explained applications of their work. Magee said:

> *Since the research here is relatively limited, what I and most of the other faculty do is-we do a lot of consulting with companies in the area. And, the idea is this is a relatively small town, a fairly rural part of (State), and so there aren't a lot of engineering firms. And so a lot of the companies around here do need engineering expertise. And so we help to provide that to companies in the area through our consulting. And then a certain amount of it is through service. You know projects like I mentioned ... I'm a member of Engineers without Borders. And so I do service projects there.*

> *Well for example, the Engineers without Borders - the three projects that we're currently working on in the (State), two of them are projects where we're actually building water distribution arrangements for cities; one in Honduras, and one in El Salvador ... In both cases they get a lot of rain for part of the year and very little rain for the rest of the year. And so we build storage tanks, usually somewhere up above the villages. And then we've got a distribution; we've figured out how to make a distribution system of pipes. And so we actually bring the water to the different villages in the area. And the idea is I use my expertise primarily to supervise a group of students. Most of the actual work is done by students at the various universities, and some of the locals in those villages.*

Richards explained his experience with Engineers without Borders as he recounted:

> *I've recently become involved in a local chapter of Engineers without Borders. Engineer without Borders is an organization that looks at ways to help developing countries and communities An example of what we've been working on is working with a community in Honduras that has ... 500 school kids in about three classrooms. For those kids we recently built a multi-classroom building for them. Actually, in collaboration with that community we're currently working on designing and planning to implement a new kind of bathroom for the school. And so this is an example of how taking my knowledge of engineering and looking for ways to apply that outside of engineering, or outside of kind of the traditional engineering environment to help serve others.*

Both Chambers and Ayers elaborated about ways that their engineering students connected to their local communities. Chambers explained:

> *I also like to work with my students to serve the ... larger community. So one example is I worked with some students during a class last spring to do a*

*semester-long service project, this academic service learning project. And they were doing things like thermal energy analysis or audit for a school building. So in that way you take some engineering understanding in a system, bring the students into that experience.*

Similarly, Ayers noted:

*I'm trying to do engineering outreach. That's one of my big areas of interest. So here at our institution we actually have a community-based project that the sophomores do as a design ... project. So I've been getting involved with that and maybe more involved with it this next year. So we do basic engineering design of various things like wheelchair ramps, or ... shelving for the library, or things like that that will then be delivered to someone in our community.*

## Communication

When academics referred to the communication aspect of transformation, they frequently mentioned the importance of tailoring communication to appropriate audiences. Among the audiences to which respondents recommended this communication be tailored included professionals who were not engineers (e.g., ophthalmologists (Craig Daniels), managers (Kevin Magee)), family (Adam Greene), peers (Sheryl Chambers), students (Sheryl Chambers, Stephanie Stahl), and the lay population (Sheryl Chambers, Stephanie Stahl, Samantha Ayers, Catrina Benson).

### *Communicating with professionals who are not engineers*
Examples of non-engineering audiences with whom engineers might engage, according to Daniels and Magee, included medical professionals and managers, respectively. Daniels explained how communication differed for an engineering journey versus a medical journey:

*So what we do is we publish the methods with a test case that we develop in engineering journals because that's the audience that we're trying - and those are in very strict engineering terms, and very rigorous, and very mathematical, and theoretical.*

*And then ... once we get the method published in an engineering journal we'll turn around and apply the method to some group of specimens or eyes or animals or whatever we use them for, and then publish the results of the work in a field-specific journal like ophthalmology.*

Magee said that engineers often know how to communicate with other engineers yet have trouble communicating with managers such that "they need to understand when they're writing something for ... a manager- They need to understand the manager's perspective. They need to understand what the manager is trying to get out of this report."

### Communicating with the public

Chambers, Stahl, Ayers, Richards, and Benson mentioned the importance of communicating one's ideas with the lay public. Richards referred to communicating information so people can understand information while also communicating that information accurately. Stahl discussed why talking to the general public is so challenging: "So the biggest challenge is understanding how to present what you do at a variety of levels ... It's relatively easy to talk to a group of experts about what you do. It is much harder to talk to a group of people who are scientifically literate but not experts in your area." Benson noted the importance of "being diverse enough to, and aware of everything that's going on in the world, and to how your research is applicable to that."

Both Chambers and Ayers made connections to engineering and policy in their responses about communication. Chambers emphasized "the importance of communicating the relevance of engineering and research work to society in general" and discussing the relevance of one's work and using "terms that they [society] can understand." Chambers explained why engineers should engage with policy makers:

> I also think that engineering PhDs should communicate a bit more with policy makers because I think that elected officials and policy makers have a limited understanding of what goes on in engineering research, and that their support is really important in our whole funding system ... So we rely a lot on government grants, and it's important that they understand what the relevance is, what the potential is of what we're doing.

Ayers elaborated about the need for engineers to connect their work to policy and to engage in cross-disciplinary activities. She referred to a recommended skill for engineers by suggesting that engineers be "well-read so that you can understand the context even in terms of policy ... governmental policy, and how what you're doing has some impact on that, or environmental impacts ... global or societal impacts."

Finally, Juan Cooke mentioned the importance of engineers breaking down complex ideas, a skill that he believed can be learned:

> Ideally they [engineers] need to be able to transfer very complex pieces of information to an audience. If you can do that, you can do anything. So, if you

*have the patience and the appreciation of so many people that's needed, and you can work yourself through that then you're in the best possible place because that means that you can, with very little effort, communicate with peers, and with a bit of effort communicate with lay people, and so anybody else in between should be an easy list.*

*So I would say that's the biggest ability, deconstructing complex arguments into simple and easy to understand language. ... It can be developed. It's not predetermined to necessarily be born with.*

## Multi-disciplinarity

Multi-disciplinarity proved to be a key aspect of transformation. This involved working with people outside one's organization (e.g., a company) or discipline to advance diversity and inclusion or to prepare students for experiences they would have after graduation (e.g., working on multi-disciplinary teams). Both Stephanie Stahl and Catrina Benson regularly interacted with colleagues and students to expand students engineering expertise. Stahl explained:

*I am very supportive of mentoring women scientists, particularly underrepresented minorities. I have a woman underrepresented minority jointly for me and another colleague, and we are working with her on developing an NIH (National Institutes of Health) postdoc - or predoctoral fellowship. I also just submitted a proposal which I'm hoping NSF (National Science Foundation) is going to fund for a woman doctoral student who's finishing up to do a post-doctoral position. Jointly, she would work at a company and it would be jointly supervised ... by me and the company scientists. So that's a real ... service area that ... ties into my professional expertise.*

Benson discussed the robotics minor at her university as a way to engage in transformation. She highlighted its contribution to students' experiences outside of their engineering major:

*But the fact that we've developed a robotics minor that's completely multi-disciplinary where we have it in such a way that students from several majors can get this minor, and they take a multi-disciplinary senior design project, which is almost unheard of, because in most schools you do a capstone experience completely in your discipline. We have outside sponsors for these projects, and we're trying to model the actual work environment that most students who graduate will go into. They're not going to go work in a cubicle with all other computer scientists, or electrical engineers, or computer engineers. So we're actually helping them to model their future workforce with this multi-disciplinary major where they're sitting in class together beyond the fresh-man year.*

*Normally they're together their freshman year because they're all in physics together, or calculus. But we now have students sitting together in their junior year taking controls.*

*We have students sitting together ... in their junior or senior year actually tak-ing controls, or taking a programming course, or taking mobile robotics, or robotics engineering. We've had companies contact us because of the way we've designed this program because they want to hire students who have this multi-disciplinary experience. And we understand that that's kind of unique.*

*You know, there are lot of schools that may have a robotics major, but once again everyone majors in robotics. Or, they may have a robotics certificate but they don't have a multi-disciplinary senior design experience. Having the stu-dents work together all the way up to graduation on a project in order to pro-duce a product where they're the domain expert on that project for that discipline. The electrical engineering student ... takes care of the electrical knowledge for whatever this project is. The CS (computer science) or software engineering [student] takes care of the programming. And the mechanical engi-neer does ... the mechanics of the system. And robotics is the perfect field for that because it's multi-disciplinary in itself.*

## Teaching

Academia respondents defined teaching as transmittal of knowledge in the classroom and outreach beyond the classroom—which has far-reaching impacts. Since teaching is a pivotal aspect of one's job as an academician, this emphasis on teaching is not surprising. Sherrie Roberts compared outcomes in industry versus academia to explain the joy that she experi-enced as an instructor:

*When you're in industry and you're working on a product ... you can see the importance of it, then I would say, that's maybe what other people see. But as far as ... how I am helping people- I think I'm helping my students and they're going to be great engineers.*

Two aspects of teaching that occurred often among academics included educating audiences outside of the traditional classroom environment and explaining nuances of teaching related to transformation. While Mark Heard, Craig Daniels, and Samantha Ayers referred to their nontraditional teaching, Mitchell Bentley expounded how he connected research to teaching in an effort to advance the engineering workforce:

> *I think the way that I do that (serve) is to include in my classes and my research a direct connection to the students, what they're working on now, and how it would be used at some point in time in the future by them or by humanity. I think that by tying everything we do for the students to a long-term goal that directly benefits society, benefits not only the students in their education process, but it also helps society because their needs are being directly seen by the students as they do the work. It further motivates the students to perform at a higher level.*

From elementary students to medical experts, Heard and Daniels translated their expertise to a broad audience. Heard described how he engaged others in, architectural acoustics. In his work with elementary school students, he prompted students' critical thinking by asking, "How does it [acoustics] work? Why does an orchestra sound this way in this hall and when somebody sings it sounds different?" Daniels explained how her expertise connected her to ophthalmology experts:

> *This year I got invited because of these publications and other things ... to serve on the faculty of the American Academy of Ophthalmology Meeting, which is a ... MD meeting for ophthalmologists. And what I did was get up and give a talk about ocular biomechanics and why it was important. But I'm one of the few PhDs that gets invited to those meetings. Because it's a continuing medical education for standard practicing ophthalmologists ... those are the kinds of things that I try to do to improve people's awareness of what we're doing and why certain aspects of glaucoma should be paid attention to with respect to clinical practice. So that's a good example of something I did very recently was serve on the faculty of this thing, give a talk to 1,000 ophthalmologists who are then going to go out and potentially change their approach, or at least hopefully it improved their understanding of glaucoma as a disease and the influence in some way their clinical practice.*

Both Linda Stephens and Ayers involved undergraduate engineering students in expertise that connected them to others outside of their classroom environment. For example, Stephens funded students to participate in a ten-week experience in France exploring global research opportunities with scientists. Ayers translated her expertise to potential women engineers and involved her undergraduate engineering students in introducing engineering to children as well. Ayers said:

*This coming year I'm starting a Society of Women Engineering chapter and we're going to do a day called (Name of Initiative) where we will go and teach elementary kids about physics and engineering. And then there's another event that I'm setting up where one of my undergraduate classes will themselves create and design demonstrations to illustrate basic engineering concepts. And then we're going to take those to a junior high group locally classroom and present those to the kids and talk a little bit about being engineers and what engineers do.*

Regarding the nuances of teaching, Chambers eloquently described what it meant to teach engineering to serve students, offered suggestions to teach engineering students, and reiterated the importance of cultivating a good learning environment for students:

*For communicating with their students I think that engineering PhDs need to understand students do not have the same technical background as their peers. And that you need to work on ... bringing them up to that level. So I think with students ... span the bridge from a lay person's terminology to very technical terms. So you're teaching them the technical terms, but you use non-technical terms to bring them there. I think with students it's also important to remember that the communication is a two-way street. So if you're standing up there and you're talking, talking, talking, and the students have no idea what you're saying then you're just wasting your breath. So it's important to check in with the students and to have their kind of active give and take with the students.*

Roberts also reflected on the benefits of her technical background in her preparation as an instructor as she shared:

*When I'm doing the prep for my classes I think having the PhD and having been exposed to sort of the hard problems ... that come up everywhere and in all different sorts of fields and subspecialties inside of electrical engineering ... that really helps me be a better teacher. And it helps me ... prepare better lectures and better material for my students. And it produces better students.*

## Industry respondents

Transformation for industry respondents encompassed a broad range of occurrence. Ways that they translated knowledge included engaging with customers, teaching in areas of outreach and company training and coaching, and applying expertise in the improvement of one's organization. Communication also emerged as respondents discussed the types of communication in which they engaged, ways to connect with an audience, and communication strategies for engineering PhD holders.

## Engaging with customers

Both Julius Kimmel and Benjamin Kinder referred to engagement with customers as key communication strategies as industry experts. Kinder noted the mandatory nature of this by saying, "I am required ... as we progress through projects, we constantly engage the customer to let them know what is going on. So, typically if it is a technical presentation we will engage the customer – sometimes I engage them up front if the problem is complex enough where I really need help to solve this." In addition to working with customers, Kimmel noted that he presented seminars and papers at conferences to expand the knowledge base in a specific area.

## Types of communication

Industry respondents communicated via e-mails, publications, and presentations. Nadine Vinson explained the critical nature of communicating in an email such that it "gets the point across in a succinct manner." Stewart Ogelsby provided insights about presentations, particularly those given at conferences. He noted that learning how to share ideas was crucial and how presentation skills were "important and paramount in every research endeavor." He went on to say that good presentation skills "improved one's conversation skills even without having a big audience." Finally, Ogelsby spelled out his publication process in industry, which allows PhD holders to publish in internal journals in the company. He discussed the diversity of these publications and how, prior to publication, the legal team at his company had to review his content.

## Connecting with your audience

Ronald Perkins, Gino Braxton, and Julius Kimmel noted the importance of connecting to an audience and offered tips for making these connections. Kimmel suggested that engineering PhD holders "try to gear your communication based on your audience ... You need to find common ground with your audience and understand a little bit about what their motives and objectives are." Perkins echoed this sentiment:

> I think they [engineering PhD holders] need to have active listening skills ... that's very important because you have to be able to understand the audience, understand what they understand, and understand what level at which you need to explain things to them for them to understand ... that's a very important characteristic.

He suggested simplifying one's vocabulary and message for an audience so they can "understand the contribution that you're making or the contribution of the deliverable that you're giving to them." Braxton reflected on the importance of being aware of an audience's perspective and tailoring messages to that audience.

## Communication strategies

Industry professionals also offered numerous strategies for communicating information. They included practice (Nicholas Poole), clear communication (Gennifer Rankin), enthusiasm for one's work (Julius Kimmel), storytelling (Nadine Vinson and Arlene Petit), prior preparation (Arlene Petit), and considering others in one's communication (Bradley Simmons).

Nicholas Poole told a story about the importance of practice in communication:

*One of the things we did in our group is that every week we would have a group meeting and that one person would have to present something at the meeting. It didn't have to be a research ... one person one time gave a presentation on the things you need to do when you're planning a camping trip. But the idea is that getting comfortable presenting in front of a group of your peers. And then developing presentations that are interesting and engaging as opposed to reading the slides.*

In his explanation of communication skills, Rankin reflected:

*Sometimes when people have a PhD ... some people misperceive them as being really, really smart, but not really knowing how to move theory into something that's practical. And I think that's really important in showing that ... you understand a lot of theory, but you actually know how to translate that into something useful.*

Using storytelling as a way to communicate was key to Vinson and Petit. While Vinson saw presentations as stories of technical work, Petit elaborated with ways to make this story comprehensible to others:

*In school we always talked about, well explain it like you were explaining it to your mother ... put yourself in somebody else's shoes who maybe isn't as familiar with your work as you are ... be able to take complicated concepts and simplify them so that they're easy to understand.*

Petit's focus on preparation countered unexpected occurrences in industry environments:

*I have a lot of meetings, and a lot times in the meetings we're projecting some-thing and I have to prepare slides, so I think being able to prepare a good pre-sentation but also have it be well rehearsed and know what you're going to say in advance, and ... be prepared ... a lot of times at work you're put in a situation where you're kind of asked things at the last minute, but you know it always helps to be prepared in advance so that you can express your story.*

Simmons highlighted differences between communication interests of technical experts with business leaders and why knowing these differences is important to engineering PhD holders:

*First, and foremost, if you were in their shoes, what is it that you would be interested in? ... if it's a peer, in all honesty the excitement's going to be gener-ated around the nuts and bolts of the technical discovery that was just made, what we learned, desire to look at the data in incredible depth, pour through it ... look at things with a fine-toothed comb. So, the technical peer is gonna' be interested ... more from a purely technical perspective, and the excitement that's generated as a result of literally what it is that we just learned.*

*The business leader, on the other hand, is going to look at that same informa-tion and expect you to be able to answer, "What are the applications of that result for my business?" It could be you've discovered a new path for making a material that's going to make my process much more environmentally friendly, for example, or it's going to make it possible for me to run at three times the rate and not have to build a new factory because I can get all the additional product that I need out of an existing line. And, it may be the same data that this technical peer was getting all excited about just because of novel looking excitements of the technology itself.*

## Teaching

Ways that industry respondents referred to teaching included university engagement (Julius Kimmel), company-sponsored outreach programs (Nadine Vinson), one-on-one engagement with engineering outreach (Nadine Vinson and Arlene Petit), application of one's work for the com-pany (Ronald Perkins), and company training and coaching (Nicholas Poole and Bradley Simmons).

### Engineering outreach

Outreach to students with current or future interests in engineering occurred via company-sponsored events and through independent efforts by industry professionals. While Vinson engaged in both company-sponsored and personal outreach, Petit connected to students independently of her company. Both Vinson and Petit volunteered with engineering organizations that reflected their demographics and values, particularly in the areas of underrepresented populations in engineering. Vinson focused on professional skills development as well as education and the engineering workforce with tutoring at her church and engaged with two student organizations:

*I try to present to the Black Grad Association and NSBE (National Society of Black Engineers) about just some career development … I've done interviewing skills, and work life hours, some time management, when I come back to try to help them gain a better understanding of some of the things you can work on while you're still in school before you get to industry or your next role.*

Petit mentioned the rewarding nature of her engagement:

*I've tried to stay really active in the community, and so on occasion I'll get involved with … the Society of Women Engineers — has a mentoring program … They have people from industry mentoring some students at the local university. And I've also done middle-school girls camp where you introduce them to engineering. So we've had a project … building a bridge or solar cars or build little airplanes. I've done a couple of those every month.*

From a company perspective, Vinson described her outreach efforts:

*For the application of the knowledge in my field to serve others, I get involved with various programs that the company actually fully supports … We have [a] science ambassador program where I go into middle schools, or even you can go into high schools, so K-12, and present whatever you want to present on how crude oil gets converted to gas, or … polymers- any topic technical that you want to present to the students to one put a face in front of them … one as a minority, to put something in front of them to see, "You can do this too." But also to just increase interest in science, and math, and engineering.*

*Another one [is] introduce a girl to engineering. So that's specifically geared towards girls and we go in and present and do hands-on experiments with them to give them a flavor on what science, and math, and females to increase those numbers.*

### Company training and coaching

Both Poole and Simmons listed coaching and training as an aspect of teaching in industry. Poole took some engineering education classes in graduate school and used that training to train interns and new people in his group "how things work." Meanwhile, Simmons focused exclusively on the development of chemical engineers within his company:

> One of the things that I was asked to give by virtue of my chemical engineering background was to actually restart and rebuild a chemical engineering function within the corporation.

> "And we hire a bunch of chemical engineers, we have several hundred. But we actually don't have a group of … practicing chemical engineers within the group. And I mean practicing traditional chemical engineering. We have a lot of people applying their skills that they learned as part of the program in non-traditional ways. So, one of the things that I'm doing is actually rebuilding that function … I've recently hired an experienced chemical engineering manager from a professional chemical industry to be my (Company Role) to pull all of that off. That's one way I'm directly applying that knowledge is one to rebuild the function. And, look at it in terms of literally down to the unit operations level. I mean looking at operations would be mission-critical to (Company). How we want to develop the expertise, and things like that. So that one's a direct application of my chemical engineering knowledge.

> The other, this goes back to the coaching and personal engagement and providing technical direction that I mentioned before, most of the mission-critical or crisis oriented assignments that … I personally choose to dive into, are the ones where I can directly apply my own chemical engineering experience either around reaction separations, you name it … but it's direct application of technical chemical engineering knowledge that I have acquired through the years. And then using that to solve problems critical to the company. At the same time, applying that same knowledge to help guide and coach less experienced engineers, chemical or otherwise, on how they might best look at and tackle a problem so that in the end they can solve it effectively as well.

## The application of knowledge, skills, findings, and insights

It is not surprising that many of the broader impacts of industry professionals were technical. These technical products included hygiene products (Gennifer Rankin), diapers and health care gowns (Benjamin Kinder), toilet paper (Benjamin Kinder), and ultrasound machines (Arlene Petit). Moreover, patents were common representations of applications of knowledge. One patent led to products that were sold for millions of dollars as storage devices while another advanced materials. Rankin elaborated on the latter, "We actually filed a patent for a new technique that could be used to aperture or put tiny holes in an elastic rubber knit material to make it breathable, which would make it more comfortable for consumers to use it."

### Application of research for organizational improvement

Ronald Perkins, Arlene Petit, and Nicholas Poole's technical expertise advanced aspects of their organizations in the areas of information systems, fiscal savings, and processes, respectively. Palmer explained the adoption of his work in his company:

> A couple of months ago I was working for a lady that was in charge of launching this new information system plant-wide. And, it doesn't actually provide us with the information that we need, nor does it allow us to communicate with our system(s) seamlessly. So, from my research, I kinda' gave her a couple of ideas … things to look out for when you know having discussions … if it isn't compatible with the system that's bad. And that's common knowledge. If you have to use too many systems to communicate and search for data that's bad. But she didn't know how bad that could be … You could have them clean stuff up but that's still, you still don't have an idea of how bad it can be once you go live. Theoretically, there are certain things that you need to pay attention to, and I just pointed a couple of those things out for her. So that was a way that I could actually apply what I've learned … through my track as a PhD to my work environment.

Poole noted that numerous aspects of his job connected to education knowledge. He developed software, did fiscal analyzes, and used control system theory to "save money within the company."

Finally, Petit presented her team's work as an example of transformation: "As a team we've been involved in basically changing a lot of the processes internally so that has been really where it was kind of recognized at the expert level for making the processes better at the company."

## Academia to industry respondents

Three areas of transformation focus for academia to industry respondents included communication, teaching, and applying knowledge. Communication presented fundamentals of effective engagement as an engineering PhD holder, along with suggestions for strengthening their communication skills.

## Communication

Blake Greiner, Virgil Sharma, and Peter Calloway identified the need for engineering PhD holders to communicate appropriately to diverse audiences. Greiner noted this as "a sensitivity to know where their audience [is], who their audience is, and where they are at mentally [and] emotionally." PhD holders also must demonstrate "an understanding of what their audience can accept and not accept and an understanding of the cultural norms of the audience."

Sharma compared communicating in industry versus academia. Mentioning communication expectations in industry, he reflected:

*Concise presentations are always much more desirable and effective than lengthy presentations in detail. They have to know their audiences if they are presenting to senior management a proposal of work solution. They have to really simplify that to the extent that it's to the point and succinct because they can easily lose their audience ... Engineers inherently don't have a good sense of that because ... sometimes they lose the audience, sometimes there is a disconnect between what they're saying and their senior management is hearing. And that can lead to frustration on both sides. So, they really need to put themselves in the shoes of the audience and adjust their communication or presentation scope accordingly.*

Calloway described the need for engineering PhD holders to be poised in their communication efforts. He expounded:

*Frequently PhD students, they kind of live at their desk, or they live in their labs, and they interact mostly with their own being with other students. But, they really need some experience presenting in front of audiences or giving talks in front of - I don't want to say hostile, but a committee or a group that may doubt their results. You know, that may be looking for something wrong. I characterize that as poise, being forceful, and articulate, and being confident in your own results. So, I've definitely seen students that have all those skills, and I've seen others that are very timid and ... they don't portray confidence.*

*An example in industry is when we present to our customers ... In our case, our customers are large customers ... they buy large quantities with each purchase, and they have very stringent expectations. So, they tend to ask hard questions, they're not always polite, sometimes they put you on the spot.*

Regarding conflicts that may arise in communication and preferred methods of communication, Calloway explained:

*It's good for PhD students to get some experience and some training in the area of communicative verbally with audiences that may not agree with them.*

*Or, maybe are motivated to disagree. And then in terms of written communica-
tion, I would say it's more learning how to be brief. What I noticed in my business and in other areas is that we rely too much on email. You know, that I
see lots of long email messages that take a long time to read, and it takes a
long time to type. And, time is very valuable. And I think a communication skill
is ... how to communicate your ideas professionally but very quickly and
briefly, and to know when to go to a phone call, or to a face-to-face meeting
... to know which medium over which to communicate is also important.*

## Teaching

Blake Greiner and Ryan Zeigler presented two unique teaching applications in their responses. While Greiner mentioned competency development as an industry application of teaching, Zeigler referred to his
parental obligation to "raise them [his children] to be problem-solver
scientists, curious about their environment and wanting to be involved."

## The application of knowledge, skills, findings, and insights

Peter Calloway told a story about the broader impacts of the company
where he worked. This company also has obtained patents. He elaborated:

*My company now is a solar power company. So we develop products that
increase the use of solar power. So one reason we've been able to hire and one
reason that people are motivated to work here is because they see all of that,
you know, the solar power in general is a good thing. It's good for society and
it's good for other people. And the necessity, electricity is a necessity and one
way to get it is solar power and it's better than other forms of power. So, the
way we apply our knowledge in an area where we think there's a commercial
benefit that there's a reasonable chance of success and that we think is a societal benefit.*

## Industry to academia respondents

Industry to academia respondents defined transformation in a variety
of ways. Some noted oral and written communication; communicating
with diverse audiences; teaching in traditional ways in a classroom; and
teaching in nontraditional ways with high school students, undergraduate
students, graduate students, and early career faculty. Furthermore, these
respondents recognized that communication can occur by applying
knowledge via technical impacts and producing patents.

## Communication

Primary areas of focus for communication included how respondents communicate and how they responded to diverse audiences. There was consensus from industry to academia professionals that engineering PhD holders should be able to organize their thoughts, articulate knowledge well verbally and in writing, and present information logically. This included projecting their voices or creating visually appealing presentations. Roland Bankston offered concise expectations about writing and distinguished differences across types of writing:

*And when they [engineering PhD holder]s write, they have to write technical writing if you want to become really effective. And when I say technical writing I mean journal paper writing, technical journal paper writing. That can be different from proposal writing for example, or other forms of writing. Because when you write a technical paper ... there are certain standards that are not the same as if you write a proposal, for example.*


*And then journal papers should be really focused, very much on conciseness, directness, 100% accuracy. No intensifiers ... no extreme adjectives like ... "excellent," or "extremely," or ... things should be really much more like a robot. Should be, "Yes, true, false, true, false," it shouldn't be ... lots of exaggerating comments. If you're going to describe your results where you're comparing them all to data, for example, you should be concrete. "The model agrees with the data within 0.01 grams/gram." ... It shouldn't be ... this is an excellent fit to data ... writing all that other crap ... doesn't work in the long run that's not the best strategy to be effective. And it also can lead to confusion and miscommunications. And then people can question your judgment. When you say that something's excellent, and then they look at it and, "I don't think it's excellent. Okay, the guy is wrong." ... it's better to have people to have trust ... in what you're saying, or what you're writing ... Stamp out ambiguity.*

### *Communicate with diverse audiences*

Eric Dillard, Randall Rice, and Terry Sherwood explained why communicating with different audiences was important. Dillard referred to the importance of realizing how detailed one should be with their audience and that they should tell a comprehensive story about their work:

*You need to understand how to communicate at different levels with different people and [understand] what their needs are. You have to know your audience.*

*So what level do you communicate on, how detailed. You know, that's the problem I see with students ... One is ... they sometimes sort of start in the middle if you will, which means they jump right in to what they want to talk about and don't set the stage for what's going on. And, I like to talk to them, I like to say that what you want to do is you want to tell a story. And so, if you're going to tell a story about your data and your research there either has to be the context or the beginning to it, and that's often missing when I see ... presentations or whatever.*

Rice focused on tailoring one's message to technical and nontechnical audiences:

*Number one characteristic is recognize not everyone is a scientist. So being able to not necessarily dumb-down what you're talking about, but taking it down to a level ... that everyone can understand. And sometimes that requires you to be able to tie it to someone that everyone can recognize, they can relate to ... sometimes I work with things and I say "Let me give you an example.*

Sherwood not only recognized the importance of tailoring information appropriately to audiences but displayed multiple levels of communication by teaching his students about the importance of differing communication across audiences:

*When I teach my classes I try to emphasize that that the people that are in a position to commit resources, whether it's money or the efforts of others, or even the freedom for you to do what you want as opposed to something else, they often have different pressures upon them and different things they're trying to satisfy. Like if you're a plant manager you're interested in safety, and labor relations, and community relations, and so forth. And if you're a marketing person you're interested in fulfilling your customer's needs at a profit. And if you're a manufacturing unit manager, you want safety and production rate and that kind of thing. And so, one of the things I stress to people is that you analyze your audience. ... they're gonna' assume that you know what you're talking about. But what they are very interested in is ... what's in it for them. And so you need to think about this.*

*And when you give talks and presentations, when you write proposals and the like, it's - you're not writing these for yourself, you're writing them to address a particular audience that may not be homogenous audience, but each element of the audience you're after you've gotta' consider how they're gonna' react ...*

*And, so the ability to analyze from different points of view what will appeal to them about what you're doing, and why what you're doing - what you're recommending should be done is a critical skill.*

Shirley Thorne explained the importance of articulating across levels as well:

*You have to articulate in a way where you can do high-level, mid-level, and low-level. You have to articulate in a way where you can communicate across those levels where you may have an audience ... that is diverse in the knowledge of engineering, or in the knowledge of the technology.*

*So you have to be able to break it down in laymen terms what the technology is trying to convey. And, be able to make it sometimes personal for your audience in terms of what the technology is doing, what it's capable of, and hopefully how it can progress what they're doing.*

*As an engineer you also have to try and meet the audience at their need. So, if you have an audience that is full of corporations, each corporation may have a specific need. And you may not be able to address all of those needs, but you have to meet some or part of the audience at their need.*

Reuben Moffit emphasized the need to engage with diverse audiences given engineering's connection to ethics, regulations, and compliance. He felt obligated to guide people as someone with 30 years of experience. He brought up how:

*It kind of helped having a PhD to kind of speak the lingo and do that. Is it because they're currently not in compliance with some laws and regulations? Is it because these are industry best practices? Is it because we know they're expanding? When they expand [is] this is the higher bar that they're going to be judged against?*

## Teaching

Although teaching was mentioned in traditional (e.g., classroom) and nontraditional ways, most teaching among industry to academia respondents extended beyond classroom teaching and included high school students, undergraduate students, graduate students, and faculty. Much of this teaching was translated as a form of mentoring or professional development.

### Traditional teaching

Eric Dillard mentioned traditional aspects of teaching and ways to be an effective teacher. His suggestions included: making analogies, putting information together in different ways, and ensuring that students comprehended material even if it was complex. Rice supported this idea of comprehension by professing, "The first thing that a person needs to understand ... If you can't do that you're not going to be able to effectively communicate your results to the broad spectrum."

### Nontraditional teaching

When it came to teaching in non-traditional settings, interviewees most often interacted with high school students, college students, and faculty. Moffit connected his teaching to policy as well.

### High school students

Philip Hays expounded regarding his community engagement with high school students, highlighting the successes and limitations working with them:

> I've had a number of high school teachers and high school students come and work in the lab in the summer. In the summer the teaching load is light so I have some time to work with them. And the high school teachers partake [in] some kind of support from the (Center Name), and they also supply some funds for the materials and supplies, so I just donate my time to work with them. I have to meet them and cover the project [so] that they can take some material back to the classroom to serve the students and maybe interest them in devices or sensors.

> And we had a high school student work with us last summer on my gas chromatography, and she built some miniature gas chromatography columns and she made a nice poster showing how these are made in clean rooms. And then she made a demonstration of liquid chromatography for the students to see in the classroom so they could see the principle of a chemical separation. So I think that was pretty successful.

> It's hard to work with a large group of high school students because ... doing research working ... one-on-one with the individual. But ... high school students come in the lab, and I usually team them up with one of the graduate students who have a project where they have measurements or data acquisition or some calculations they're doing with the data so that students can do some work with them in the lab.

*And we did have a student who [was] coauthor on a paper a couple of years back where he was helping one of my graduate students measure the characteristics of a microvalve.*

## Undergraduate students

Randall Rice deeply reflected on his contribution to the development of undergraduate engineering students beyond teaching them in courses. His big picture perspective drew upon his experience as an engineering PhD holder such that he anticipated what students might need to do to achieve success as engineers later in their careers:

*At the undergrad level ... I'm helping them to develop their own research skills and their own research prowess. Being able to look at a problem and see ... "Do the results make sense?" ... 'cause a lot of students come in, undergrads having no research background. So having to ... sow those seeds within them early so that they can go forward and then get comfortable, actually giving them a little small research problem, design their experiments, carry out their experiments, get the results, and then take the time to sit down and analyze the results. To understand ... "Does this seem valid? Does the data I have correspond or correlate well with what's been published before?"*

*And so, when I meet with the students I know I can see different things that they need or they should do to go through the experiences I had. So, in that aspect it is valuable because I know where they're going and I know what they're going to need. And so I wouldn't want somebody in my position that didn't know that because then you could send the student on a wrong direction.*

## Graduate students

Roland Bankston and Aaron Whitehurst identified their engagement with graduate students as important aspects of transformation. Bankston explained:

*When I meet with graduate students on research, a very large fraction of that, probably at least 80% ... is really education rather than ... research. What I mean by that is that a lot of it I'm just teaching them how to think ... I'm pointing them to different ... research areas, different fields that you can learn stuff about. I am, deriving models with them. So a lot of that work is ... trying to educate them to a level that they can progress on the research. So it's a pretty heavy teaching mission even though technically most people would that on the research ... I would put that as at least 80% on the teaching side.*

Whitehurst also described his commitment mentoring graduate students:

> Because of my knowledge I can mentor them [graduate students] to learn and grow in a highly technical area. And so I can influence them becoming successful, independent researchers or problem-solvers ... launching on their own careers whether it's academics, or in industry, or in government laboratories.

### Early career faculty

Aaron Whitehurst identified mentoring of his colleagues as another form of teaching, "I've been in position to actively mentor for a number of younger faculty members. And I think in many cases have been able to provide sought after advise or ... hopefully act as a positive influence on some younger colleagues."

### Non-academics

Reuben Moffit described his connection to government as an engineering PhD holder:

> And even in the latter stages of my career, when I got involved here with (University) was actually to put on a seminar in Washington where we invited a whole cross section of bureaucrats and got together industry experts, and it was amazing to me that these folks had never been in the same room before, to put on a two-day, very high powered seminar in some very technical areas so we could make it clear to the regulators and other bureaucrats in Washington what is the state of the art in this area.

## The application of knowledge, skills, findings, and insights

Ways that industry to academic respondents have applied knowledge, skills, findings, and insights included consulting with other companies, and patenting.

### *Broader impacts (technical)*

Engineering is one part of a larger system that produces projects within companies and organizations. As such, respondents often mentioned a specific application of their work. Roland Bankston told a story about the application of his technology development, resulting in billions of dollars of revenue for companies and increased product quality and throughput:

> And so a lot of the technology I have developed ... has been used and is used on real pharmaceutical compounds to ... make higher quality pharmaceuticals

*and to make them cheaper basically; focusing more on quality and reliability . . .
to making sure that you produce the same drug or compound, or the same structure every time . . . That's had a pretty big impact on society and humanity.*

*Because I'm usually not told what the drug compound is . . . I'm not allowed to
tell anyone so what it means is it's hard for me to get exact number [of] esti-
mates of how many processes my technology's been applied to. But it's probably in the billions − billions of dollars per year.*

*. . . I have contributed to a process that made compounds that . . . are proba-
bly in the billions of dollars per year if you put all the compounds . . . pharmaceutical compounds together. But of course a lot of people have also
contributed to those processes too.*

Bankston expressed how he might engage in a process, particularly the
de-bottlenecking process:

*So then they will call me in and then I will give them a bunch of - but these
are their technical problems. And the technical problems are such that I don't
need to know the molecular structure of the compound to understand the
problem. And then I'll come back and I'll say, "These are things that I would try,
you know, that you should look into." So, "Take this measurement. If it gives
you this it tells you that you should try this. If the measurement tells you
this you should try this. If you try this particular technology, that maybe I didn't
develop maybe somebody else developed, if you try this other technology." So I
give them, you know, different ideas of experiments to gain information that
will - or technologies that they should use to de-bottleneck their process.*

*But also as my research, some of that research, a non-trivial amount, is with
companies. These are primarily pharmaceutical companies. And so a lot of the
technology I have developed is used, has been used and is used, on real pharmaceutical compounds to . . . make higher quality pharmaceuticals and to
make them cheaper basically; focusing more on quality and reliability . . . making sure that you produce the same drug or compound, or the same structure
every time .*

Aaron Whitehurst discussed how his work has influenced optical tele-
communication and has led to a field of products that have been adopted
in telecommunications. He professed "that infrastructure . . . has impact
on anybody . . . who depend(s) on high-speed communications . . . This
was a very . . . general purpose technology and so others realized this

technology could be useful into laser-controlled chemical reactions. There's a lot of people using my technology for that kind of work."

Terry Sherwood offered a chemical-related industry safety example, as he stated:

*"... In the chemical related industry ... there's several aspects of it. Of course some of the things you do are going to help people's lives and so forth in general. But, in a more specific sense safety is very, very important. And in (Company) all managers spent a good percentage of their time and effort trying to make sure that nobody was going to get hurt, or the plant wasn't going to burn down, or boil up, or whatever, and so you were trying to figure out how people could do unusual, non-repetitive things involving chemistry safely.*

*Like one of the things that we made as an intermediate chemical, in the process I worked on was hydrogen cyanide. So if you're going to make a couple hundred million pounds a year of hydrogen cyanide you've got to consider what the potential for that kind of thing might be if it got out, or leaked, or polymerized, or something like that. Youre always working with hazardous things ... You didn't pass it off to a safety person. If you were a manager you were responsible. And you were responsible for your own people and for your customers, and your operations, and everything else.*

Finally, Shirley Thorne mentioned the broader impacts of her work:

*In my particular field applying the knowledge that we gain from materials to help with sustainable environments, applying those materials to alternative energy sources ... applying different materials to understanding biological and bioengineering devices. And so all of these things are directly related back to the community and how with engineers we of course are - are here to serve the community and to make life better at least that's the way I see it, for not only the national but the international community. So having a global perspective in terms of how we serve a global community.*

Mark Winkler and Philip Hays connected their work to patents. Hays presented detail about his work and the patent process:

*We had to design a valve for a fuel cell. And so the sponsor wanted us to make this valve as small and as low power as possible. And valves up to that point had been made with separate components that are assembled. And so with my graduate student we came up with a design where we could integrate the actuator coil and the fluid flow channels onto a single substrate. And we filed a patent on that. ... we first filed an invention disclosure on that. And then we built it here, built first the actuator, and then we built the actuator with the flow channel; demonstrated its performance. And the patent was granted.*

## So what?

Compared to other stewardship codes, *transformation* came up most frequently among interviewees, even in responses to questions focused solely on generation and conservation. Respondents were eager to discuss ways that they communicated their work and offered numerous suggestions for engineering PhD holders to communicate effectively.

Academics confirmed that they were expected to communicate broadly as engineering PhD holders. They did not have the luxury of working only with people in their current disciplinary areas or even in academia. Examples of external (non-academic) collaborators included industry sponsors and researchers. Teaching did not occur only in university classrooms but also among K-12 students and to experts out of one's discipline. How a respondent taught was addressed along with an awareness of how to provide the optimal environment for learning. Broader impacts of technical work and of outreach were mentioned as a subset of teaching.

Industry respondents mentioned clients as key stakeholders with whom they had to communicate. They emphasized that everyday communication was vital, including e-mails. Tailoring one's communication to an audience was a success strategy as an engineering PhD holder working in industry. Many industry professionals reiterated details about ways to communicate well, including telling good stories and being outward focused for communication. Teaching examples in industry included outreach to universities and students and internal training in one's company. Applications of knowledge aligned closely with the industry in which one worked.

Communication was a recurring theme among industry to academia and academia to industry respondents. Academia to industry audiences echoed the necessity of tailoring one's communication appropriately for customers and for audiences that might not want to know intricate technical details or might not agree with them. Furthermore, industry to academia respondents also mentioned the importance of communication repeatedly and the need to respond appropriately to diverse audiences. A reason for this communication related directly to ethics and compliance as engineers. Teaching expanded to engagement with high school students, undergraduate students, graduate students, early career faculty, non-academics, and representatives from other companies. Technical work and patents represented many of the contributions of industry to academia respondents.

## Students

- See Berdanier et al. (2016) for a blueprint for graduate students' development of transformation.

## Faculty

- Reflect upon ways that your technical work translates to diverse audiences and environments, particularly in the classroom.
- Develop different versions of your research story for various audiences: long versions (i.e., for technical audiences) and short versions (i.e., for laypersons). Practice delivering both versions and gather feedback about the quality of your communication and comprehension by the audience of your work.
- Explore and communicate the implications of your work so people outside your lab and environment can connect your work to broader society, policy, and decision-making.

## Industry professionals

- Form partnerships with universities to introduce students to industry work and how their work can be applied outside of their research laboratories.
- Practice succinct communication that tailors your technical expertise to diverse audiences.
- Identify ways to translate and share your expertise to teach, train, and coach others in your organization who may benefit from your knowledge. This knowledge also might be used to enhance processes and advance internal communication in your organization.

## References

Berdanier, C. G. P., Tally, A., Branch, S. E., Ahn, B., & Cox, M. F. (2016). A strategic blueprint for the alignment of doctoral competencies with disciplinary expectations. *International Journal Of Engineering Education*, *32*, 1759–1773.

Golde, C. M., & Walker, G. E. (2006). *Envisioning the future of doctoral education: Preparing stewards of the discipline, Carnegie essays on the doctorate.* San Francisco, CA: Jossey-Bass.

# PART III

# What Do Engineering PhD Holders Do?

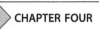

# CHAPTER FOUR

# Characteristics and expectations

*I always tell students that graduate school is more like a baseball batting aver-age than it is like a basketball free throw percentage. What I mean by that like (is that) a good baseball batting average is 33%. A good basketball free throw percentage is 90%. You have to be willing to take the seven misses to get the three hits. As a graduate student, you have to be somewhat tenacious because you're gonna' have a lot of misses to get a hit.*

**Mark Winkler, PhD, Department Chair**

Winkler used a sports analogy to emphasize the importance of persis-tence as a characteristic needed for engineering PhD holders to be success-ful. The concept of persistence came up as both a characteristic and expectation of engineering PhD holders.

This chapter reports responses of engineering PhD holders to two interview questions: (1) Within your work environment, what is expected of you as an engineering PhD, and (2) What are the most important knowledge, skills, norms, attributes, ideas, questions, or perspectives that an engineering PhD should possess? After completing and analyzing all interviews, the research team compiled 88 characteristics (Appendix 2) and 92 expectations (Appendix 3) that respondents identified regarding ideal attributes of engineering PhD holders.

The first question focused primarily on *expectations*, which highlighted academia or industry's expectations of respondents' personal roles and responsibilities as engineering PhD holders during a typical work day (e.g., interactions or work hours). The second question aligned with *char-acteristics*, which referred more broadly to the knowledge, skills, and pro-fessional or personal attributes of any engineering PhD holder. Although expectations and characteristics are closely related, expectations were *per-formed in a specific context* while characteristics *transcended a specific work envi-ronment* and were more general.

*Demystifying the Engineering PhD.*
DOI: https://doi.org/10.1016/B978-0-12-801593-3.00004-9

## Characteristics

Since characteristics transcend environments, many responses to the interview questions about knowledge, skills, norms, attributes, ideas, questions, or perspectives aligned with Golde and Walker's (2006) definition of stewardship, thereby confirming the prevalence of stewardship as a characteristics of engineering PhD holders. Of the three stewardship tenets (i.e., generation, conservation, and transformation), academia respondents reported highest occurrences of transformation and generation, industry and academic to industry respondents connected most to transformation and conservation, and academia to industry respondents most often professed transformation and generation. In addition to generation, conservation, and transformation, other top characteristics included persistence (academia); problem solving (industry and industry to academia); and work ethic (academia to industry).

## Academia respondents

Academia respondents identified transformation, generation, and persistence as the characteristics most needed of engineering PhD holders. The aspect of transformation that dominated responses related to communicating information to others in a variety of ways. Generation required that respondents demonstrate competence about ways their work could advance engineering knowledge. Persistence arose as a characteristic needed to continue the work of one's field despite potential challenges facing engineering PhDs, who are often expected to be technical visionaries.

### Transformation

Aspects of transformation identified as a characteristic by academia respondents related to communication, which included being able to break complex ideas into simple ones, writing well, speaking well, and tailoring content to an audience. Christopher Roe and Mark Heard recognized differences across writing genres and mentioned the importance of communication across modes. Roe explained that "it's different to write a paper than it is to write other things like letters and poetry, and writing a proposal is a very different skill compared to writing a paper." To get quality research done, Heard recommended that engineering PhD holders move beyond writing articles and giving technical presentations to "communicating within your own research group or with collaborators." Heard also highlighted why understanding one's own work is not enough in terms of communication and why breaking complex ideas down into simple ones is important. He advised against "rambling on too much" recommended  "knowing your audience" and not "dumbing everything down." He suggested a few questions for engineering PhD holders to ask: "What do people want to know about what I'm doing? Why do they want to know it? How am I going to explain this clearly?"

Adam Greene, Catrina Benson, Darnell Baker, and Sherrie Roberts identified the need to communicate information beyond one's area of technical expertise and presented almost identical statements about the importance of translating information that may be common with non-technical audiences. Several respondents offered advice to facilitate this translation. Roberts suggested "putting yourself in the position of the audience" or "continuing in your life to interact even socially with people of a variety of different backgrounds" in an effort to "communicate with all sorts of different people." Mitchell Bentley said that engineering students and faculty should practice their communication skills no matter how well they think they communicate. Baker mentioned that most people's parents are not scientists or don't have an engineering background so "How would you explain something to your parents or to your friends who are not engineers?" Greene referred to this as "an ability to describe complicated things accurately but in a way that somebody else can understand." He provided another perspective:

> You need to be able to adjust to the audience . . .. it's easy to talk to your peers where you use differential equations . . . But it's probably more important to be able to communicate difficult technical things in a way that other people can understand.

> . . . It could be your boss, or your boss's boss's boss who you know probably knows as much technically as you do, but he doesn't have the time to get all the details. So you have to be able to describe to him . . . what the issues are in a way that he can understand without using a bunch of equations . . . to distill the key things, technical things . . . with relatively simple words.

> . . . That's a skill you also need if you're talking to a customer . . . a salesman or something, you've got a product and you need to be able to indicate how

*great your idea is, and how great your product is in words that a non-technical person can understand.*

*You have to have those skills if you're talking with media. You know lots of times engineers are gonna' have to talk on television, or a newspaper, and you've gotta' be able to make sure that the reporter understands what the issues are and will properly convey those in his report ... You can't just snow him with a bunch of equations.*

Benson echoed Greene's thoughts:

*I think an important trait, just thinking about the grants I've gotten funded, is being able to take a technical subject and communicate to a layman exactly what it is you want to do and why it's something they should care about ... That's key to being able to do the research because if you're doing this really, really cool high level research but no one understands it enough to appreciate it, then what's the point? And I think as an engineer one of our goals is to use science and math to design something to make the world a better place.*

*And so designing this better device or object doesn't mean anything if no one understands what it's for and how to use it. So I think being able to do research at that level ... you have to be grounded in your research, make it reasonable. You can't get to the point where you say "I'm doing something so high level it doesn't matter if anyone understands it."*

## Generation

Generation as a characteristic related to asking the right questions, understanding the fundamentals of a discipline, and creating new knowledge in that field. Asking questions is important because questions often lead to advancement in one's field. Mark Heard said that "sometimes being able to understand how to ask a question is actually just as important as knowing how to solve it." He suggested asking, "How do we best evaluate - or how do we best tackle the problem?" Samantha Ayers believed PhD holders should ask, "What question do you want to answer? How are you going to answer it? What graph are you going to present that's going to provide evidence for that question?"

Being a scholar involves paying attention to details, having vision, and understanding fundamental principles. Heard asserted that "understanding those (fundamental) principles really gives you a lot of insight to interpret results correctly." Regarding being a scholar, Adam Greene posited that scholars must do research to advance knowledge: "If you're gonna' be a professor, you've gotta' be a scholar. You've gotta' know your area. You've gotta' know it cold. And you've gotta' be advancing it." For Sherrie Roberts, scholars know how to "think about very difficult problem, not just the problems that your teacher gives you." He reiterated "working on very big hard problems that nobody's ever done before," "applying something new to a different area and ... bringing in people who haven't looked at it before," and "working on something that is honestly important." Roberts also explained how someone might determine if their work is making an impact:

*I see so much getting published that is just sort of a delta change on what somebody else did and where the importance argument is quite weak. The impact argument is quite weak. It doesn't necessarily have to be a practical impact, but it can be an impact that advances understanding of something. But I think a lot of it is just small stuff. And so I think that's something very important for PhDs to understand their work in the context of sort of their field and other fields, and feel that you're doing something which they think will have a decent impact and it isn't just publishing to publish.*

Craig Daniels explained why having a research vision that is informed from knowledge of one's field is imperative for engineering PhD holders:

*You have to understand the broader field and how your work in particular fits into the broader field and why it's important. That tells you of the 50 different ways you can approach a research project which of the ways you should do it and how you should use the results to push science forward. That's where vision comes in.*

To demonstrate this expertise, Christopher Roe offered multiple suggestions:

*You need to be methodical, systematic. You need to be very careful at documenting what you're doing. You need to be aware of what the norms are ... what the typical standards of rigor in your field; what's expected. And that means, for example, if you do experiments, be familiar with the limitations and advantages of different experimental techniques.*

## Persistence

Another characteristic identified by academia respondents was perseverance or persistence, which was exemplified by overcoming failure, maintaining focus, staying patient, remaining determined, and being curious. Linda Stephens defined this as an ability to "continue despite roadblocks." Regarding failure and persistence, Craig Daniels noted:

*To succeed in ... research-related engineering you have to be tenacious because even with good vision and creativity you can't ever give up ... that's why they call it research because you're constantly researching for the answer. You never find it the first time ... you'll try something and fail and learn something and then try a new approach and fail. And then do a little bit more research and try another approach and fail ... The fourth or fifth time you'll get it right and make some progress.*

Sheryl Chambers echoed this perspective by mentioning the importance of being "fully committed to following through" with research to maintain rigor. In addition to curiosity and focus, she emphasized "not giving up" and knowing that these attributes are needed "beyond just being smart and ... knowing your field." Mitchell Bentley suggested that engineering PhDs have "a focus and a mindset on looking at a problem that they're trying to solve." He reflected that "so often people can become distracted in all of the side paths that research can take them down."

## Industry respondents

Industry respondents identified transformation, conservation, and problem-solving skills as the most important characteristics engineering PhD holders should possess. Transformation consisted of demonstrating effective communication skills such that information could be shared effectively with audiences outside engineering. Remaining characteristics aligned closely with technical competence, namely mastering engineering fundamentals via conservation, and knowing how to solve ambiguous technical problems given user-defined constraints.

### Transformation

Numerous respondents identified written communication (Julius Kimmel, Nadine Vinson, Nicholas Poole, and Gennifer Rankin), verbal communication (Julius Kimmel, Nadine Vinson, Gennifer Rankin, and Arlene Petit), and general communication skills (Nicholas Poole, Benjamin Kinder, Arlene Petit, Gino Braxton, and Bradley Simmons) as imperative for engineering PhD holders.

### *Communication skills*

Although Kimmel, Poole, and Rankin spoke generally about the importance of written skills for engineering PhD holders, Vinson added that it was important to comprehend technical concepts with the ability to write about those concepts thoroughly. Poole also mentioned that he recognized the importance of writing from personal experience.

Rankin, Kimmel, and Vinson explained how oral communication skills are pivotal for effective presentations. Rankin noted that such skills are applicable across all engineering disciplines, while Kimmel focused on the importance of presentation skills for oral communication "both at a deep level and at a high level." Vinson provided insight about how presentation skills applied to both technical and nontechnical audiences since an audience may "not really familiar with all of the kind of details of how something works."

In addition to written and oral communication skills, industry respondents discussed communication more broadly. Poole noted that clear communication increased productivity and enhanced clarity in the workplace and makes one a "very valuable commodity." Kinder suggested that engineering PhD holders craft an elevator speech:

> It's the ability to boil down highly technical problems down to very basic principles that anybody can understand. That is very important especially if I am talking to a salesperson trying to explain to him how difficult it is to commercialize a particular material- if I'm too technical I won't get it across ... I've got to boil the details down to how is it impacting him.

### Sharing information with non-engineering audiences

In his citation of technical curiosity as a characteristic needed of an engineering PhD holder, Bradley Simmons noted the importance of engineers driving and delivering the needs of business with "the ability to ... translate that curiosity and knowledge into effective solutions, meaning being able to sort the academically interesting from the practical," resulting in "the ability to sell management on those ideas so that you can gain funding and/or time to keep the work going." He candidly admitted that "a lot of our PhDs really struggle to be able to do that. Bright technically; can't relay their ideas very well." He elaborated:

> One of the things I see as a shortcoming of a lot of our folks is that they're very savvy technically but can't speak in such a way that is actually appropriate to the level of the audience that they're addressing. And, a lot of our PhD, particularly in the R&D setting, will speak to senior management in much the same way as they would speak to a technical peer and, that V.P. is looking for the elevator speech, not the two-hour detailed mechanistic explanation of that last experiment that you ran. So, tailoring communications and being able to really

*explain what one is doing to a variety of different backgrounds and audiences is very important.*

Gino Braxton also confirmed the importance of engineers translating technical information in practical ways outside technical circles:

*Equally important is the ability to articulate those concepts in a manner that others can easily understand. So, with a PhD we often get ourselves so down in the weeds, and we like to talk in the weeds in great detail and explain ... and show our knowledge in it. Unless we can really explain to a business executive what it is we're talking about and what that value really is that they can appreciate and understand then I think we've really failed. I would really expect a PhD to be able to do that kind of work as well. It comes back to the ability to take those complicated ideas and concepts and be able to translate them into an understandable narrative that explains the research.*

Aligned with Braxton's suggestion for the development of a narrative, Arlene Petit referred to the importance of storytelling such that engineers combine both technical and communication skills:

*It's not always just about getting your results, but you have to be able to put together a story and tell it to your audience so that they understand what you did ... I think you have to have good synthesis skills ... You have to be able to interpret your data and results and then communicate them properly.*

## Conservation

Comprehending fundamental engineering concepts and knowing how to obtain pertinent information closely align with conservation. Julius Kimmel, Stewart Oglesby, and Gino Braxton described this as having a "mastery of engineering fundamentals," knowing your subject, and understanding "first principles," respectively. To do this, Kinder suggested that engineering PhD holders be "pretty open" to acquiring information, be "go-getters," and "branch out" of industry to academia and national labs.

Respondents offered detailed examples of fundamentals. Kimmel recommended that engineers demonstrate competence in statistics and analysis tools such as Minitab. Ronald Perkins suggested mastery of the scientific method, understanding of a methodology and analyses (i.e., quantitative and qualitative), having an ability to critique, and knowing the importance of information and its relevancy. Braxton professed that any engineering PhD program and degree should provide the following:

*It's certainly a deep understanding and appreciation for the value of mathematics in modeling- understanding of the physical nature of variability ... Also the foundational engineering components of just engineering analysis, problem recognition, problem statement, candidate solutions, and looking through those kinds of solutions to select the best solution.*

## Problem-solving skills

The ability for engineering PhD holders to problem solve resonated with many industry respondents. While Gennifer Rankin recommended that engineering PhD holders possess strong problem solving abilities, Kimmel labeled this problem solving ability "fundamental understanding of how to go about evaluating and solving real-world problems." Gino Braxton supported engineering PhD holders' abilities to "look at things systemically and in an overall manner" to articulate problems and identify solutions. He further connected problem solving to comprehension of foundational engineering concepts such as engineering analysis, problem recognition, and problem statements, highlighting the importance of engaging with these concepts while seeking an optimal solution.

Several respondents expounded about the problem solving process. Benjamin Kinder spoke about the patience required in a problem solving process and highlighted mistakes that many people make, including not being patient enough to fix a solution one step at a time. Ronald Perkins offered concrete advice about how to problem solve via the ability to ask questions and to create a timeline:

*... You want to be able to break your questions into problems, methodology, and a success matrix. If you can do that you can essentially create whatever knowledge you want to from making sure you ask questions ... the most important characteristic is being able to ask the right questions ... Sometimes people jump to the conclusion of what's the solution rather than ... a problem. And these questions need to be asked in order to understand the problem.*

Bradley Simmons reflected on the problem solving process for engineering PhD holders in his company and noted that problem solving should closely align with the needs of the company:

*They need to be able to think ... multiple steps ahead. I see too many PhDs that run their research program literally an experiment at a time, and they don't think in terms of, "Okay, when I run this experiment, one, what question am I actually trying to answer? Two, is the experiment itself properly designed to answer that question? Three, what are the possible results that I could get from this experiment. Depending on the result what direction would I go?"*

*Which is where I get into thinking ahead a little bit as opposed to allowing the last result to dictate where you go next. Which is kind of a shorthand way of saying that the PhDs need to have a strategy around which they're actually try-ing to do their discovery, or plan their problem solving. And ... four ... focus on the problems which if ... solved, will generate results that are of interest to the corporation ... either for a product, things that would improve what the corporation is doing today, or provide valuable building blocks for businesses or technologies the company might choose to pursue in the future.*

## Academia to industry respondents

Academia to industry respondents identified transformation, conser-vation, and work ethic as the characteristics most needed of engineering PhD holders. Although transformation and conservation responses mir-rored other responses across sectors, work ethic emerged exclusively given the fast pace of industry. As such, a strong work ethic, coupled with tech-nical knowledge, was identified by academia to industry respondents who compared academic and industry experiences of engineering PhD holders.

## Transformation

The communication aspect of transformation resonated with academia to industry respondents. In addition to having a desire to get something done and possessing technical competency, Blake Greiner claimed that even making eye contact sets an engineering PhD holder apart from others:

*Do they look me in the eye when they talk about things? Because if they can't look me in the eye immediately, they can't tell me bad news, they can't tell me good news, they can't talk to other people ... They need to be able to get up and present in front of a group of people. They need to be able to talk to peo-ple and defend their ideas.*

Ryan Zeigler declared that PhD holders must understand "that there are a variety of audiences and that your message needs to be tailored to those audiences." He expounded:

*I think it would be useful for any PhD student to have maybe more experiences, or at least some educational background in technical communication because I happened to have a really good education before I got to (University) and so I didn't need to learn how to write when I got there. But I know a lot of engineers don't know how to write. They don't know how to do public speaking. We're trying to do more of that in the undergraduate, but again, when you get to the PhD there's a whole new level. You know, you've got the highest degree that's granted. There's some expectation that you're going to be a leader and to be the person who has to make the presentations to wide audiences. And so, some sort of background in that area, some kind of things that are beyond the technical skills, the people skills so that you can read audiences and know that they need a different way of conveying the message that you want to get across ... I don't know exactly how you do that, but you know it kinda' gets to if we're graduating PhDs and they're going to go be professors, well you should have some training for those skills that don't involve just being an expert in the technical area. You know, how do you actually teach a class? How do you manage TAs? How do you run a research program? So I could see some technical communication and maybe some project management, business-type skills.*

## Conservation

Blake Greiner and Ryan Zeigler both listed conservation as a characteristic of engineering PhD holders in the form of technical expertise. Greiner placed much of the responsibility for a PhD student's development and competency on a research advisor:

*And the technical competency, that's really left up to the advisor or the subject matter that they're in. There's probably some key items that need to be considered overall ... Do they have good statistics, do they have the math, are they getting a fundamental enough education to be able to grow and develop throughout their whole career rather than just learning how to solve one particular problem that their advisor taught them how to solve?*

Ziegler offered another perspective by eloquently comparing the need for engineering PhD holders to distinguish between engineering's structured problems (which he refers to as discipline) and ambiguous problems (which he refers to as freeform):

*I think there's a balance that needs to be between discipline and freeform. There needs to be some discipline to know that there's an impasse that you're going toward and to keep a focus. But if everything's discipline ... nothing new ever happens. So there needs to be an explicit balance between the discipline of ... "I have problems that need to be solved, I have defined an area, and we're going to stay within these boundaries." But then an ability to turn that discipline off at the appropriate times to go beyond the rigidity of those walls to build the new knowledge, to pull pieces of things together across traditional boundaries.*

## Work ethic

Blake Greiner and Peter Calloway highlighted the importance of engineering PhD holders having a strong work ethic. Greiner called this "a fire in the belly" and having a "desire to get stuff done." Calloway combined work ethic and determination as positive engineering PhD characteristics. He noted that earning a PhD was an automatic reflection of one's technical competency and that a strong work ethic made someone stand out. He said,

> By the time somebody had finished a PhD they'd proven that they have the basic intelligence to solve those problems. But, as you might know in academia, or as a PhD student, some people work really hard and want to finish quickly and do a great job, and others just kind of tread water ... They kind of work on what they feel like doing when they feel like doing it. And it can take six or seven years or something to finish their PhD.

> And so, when I'm hiring, I'm always looking for somebody-their attitude ... Once I see they have a doctorate or a Master's degree, or they have some experience ... I assume that their technical credentials are good. But, I'm really looking more for how would they work in a team. Will they work as hard as everybody else? Will they set a good example? I'm looking for their ability to adapt and to deliver on a deadline.

He further highlighted the differences in work ethic expectations between academic and industry environments:

> One thing about academia is it moves very slow (sic) and it has its own pace ... most deadlines are extendable, and if they're missed there aren't really dire consequences. ... In my business we have to do stuff on time or we lose money.

## Industry to academia respondents

Mirroring industry to academia respondents identified transformation, problem-solving skills, and conservation as the characteristics most needed of engineering PhD holders. Respondents expected engineering PhD holders to communicate well, to demonstrate technical expertise, and to know how to find answers to problems even if these answers were not readily available. In sum, engineering PhD holders were expected to operate at the highest levels of proficiency in their organizations.

## Transformation

Roland Bankston, Aaron Whitehurst, and Philip Hays disclosed the importance of clear written and oral communication. While Bankston emphasized utilizing these skills at both the Bachelor's and the PhD levels, Whitehurst cited the importance of doctoral-level written and oral communication skills so one's success is not limited.

Both Whitehurst and Randall Rice discussed the importance of engineers tailoring their communication to their audiences so that a student at any educational level, or even family members, could comprehend technical content. They confirmed that *how* a message is communicated was just as important as the message itself if a goal was to retain the interest of the people with whom engineers were communicating. Whitehurst stated:

*Depending on the audience there might be . . . more detailed communication. But in many cases whether it's a manager, or whether it's the general public, they're not going to pay any attention to, or allow you to launch onto a long detailed dissertation without capturing their interest . . .. boiling down what's important about what I have to say, and saying it clearly and quickly. . . is important to capture people's attention.*

Rice talked about the value of engineers dissecting problems and then being able to communicate solutions of the problem to anyone. This, coupled with one's technical proficiency, confirmed the proficiency of a good engineer:

*One of the things I think an engineering student should have, or an engineering PhD should have is the ability to take any problem, whatever it is, and be able to break that problem down, and then be able to disseminate and . . . with clarity explain the problem, or solution to that problem to anyone. I don't care whether they're a PhD or not. Being able to clearly explain the solution to a problem at anyone at any level really shows how well a PhD student or that PhD engineer has developed themselves. Because I should be able to go to . . . an undergrad right now, or go to someone outside, even my own parents, and explain what I'm doing right now, and they understand it. And they do. My dad understands exactly what I'm doing. And my dad just has a management degree. So, you're not just learning to be a scientist . . . as an engineering PhD. You also need to take your engineering skills and be able to use those skills to help others understand.*

Rice appreciated industry's broad, big picture thinking outside of science and industry's focus on linking engineering applications to current trends. He noted stereotypes about engineers and how they communicated the application of science and engineering:

> A lot of times people misunderstand that engineers are mistaken for scientists because we're so caught up in the nitty-gritty of the science. But at the same time I'm also thinking, "How do I make it better? How do I improve upon it? How is it applicable?" ... Engineers are more application-based instead of just pure science-based. And that's one of the things I always look at when I talk to other engineering PhDs ... I find out they're so ingrained in the science behind it that they forget well how do we explain it to engineering students.

Terry Sherwood corroborated the responses of Whitehurst and Rice "If I hadn't had all of that technical preparation and also communications ... I wouldn't have been able to do a good job."

Mark Winkler emphasized the importance of articulation and the definition of articulation within an engineering context:

> It's one thing ... to see a problem, but to with that problem, to be able to articulate a solution. Now, "articulate it" can mean different things. It could be a schematic. It could be a mathematical model. It could be a prototype. It could be an operation improvement ... I like to use the word "articulate" because it's in some ways your performance in engineering school that you're gonna' need to articulate.

## Problem-solving skills

The possession of problem-solving skills was both an explicit and an implicit expectation of many engineers and of the engineering profession. Many industry to academia respondents prided themselves on the ability to solve problems and to move engineering forward.

Several respondents operationalized problem solving across various contexts and discussed what it meant to be a problem solver. Roland Bankston strongly professed that problem-solving skills were the foundation for engineering, which does not always have prescribed tools readily available for use. He said:

> If someone doesn't have that [problem-solving skills], they're pretty useless ... If you don't have that you can't draw a connection, and typically most problems today are pretty sophisticated. So there isn't typically a single tool you pick up on the shelf, and bam, it solves it ... or if there is a tool that solves it it's not obvious what the tool would be immediately unless you have a really strong knowledge of a bunch of tools.

Philip Hays added that problem-solving skills must accompany analytical thinking because "at the PhD level there's more than just analytical capability, because you need to be ready to think of different ways to solve a problem." He added:

> One of the important things that the students learn is how to dissect a problem into its component parts and then do a controlled experiment ... whether it's an experiment in the lab or just a modeling where they're looking at a specific set of variables to dissect the problem and analyze which are the critical aspects that need to be studied to improve or solve ... make a better device, a better design, or understand the physics better. It's important to be systematic in terms of analyzing and then thinking about the different pieces of the problem and seeing what experiments you can do or what modeling you can do to get a better understanding of what's happening.

Terry Sherwood shared his mindset of solving open-ended, complex problems. He highlighted a need to not be intimidated by problems that have not been solved before and to develop the ability to frame, solve, and avoid problems if possible. He noted the importance of anticipating potential problems that might arise:

> You need to have the ability to look at how what you're doing might affect or be affected by other operations. And you have to look into the future and try to anticipate what the difficulties might be and how you can either avoid them or solve them quickly if they arise ... If you know the kinds of things that can go wrong and where the problems are likely to be then you can look at what you're trying to achieve at the instant, but you have to look more broadly and time wise and so forth to say, "What are the end results I want and how can I get there most effectively?"

Reuben Moffit expressed strong views about the connection of problem solving abilities to engineering via a comparison of science, technology, and engineering:

> When an engineer hires on, the reason they have a degree that says engineering at the end, and it doesn't say science at the end, and it doesn't say technology at the end, is because these folks are used to working with data and solving problems with numbers ... They don't put their fingers up in the air and see which way the wind is blowing ... they're not ... looking at public opinion necessarily, they're looking at facts. And they get data. And, they know how to correlate data and basically solve problems with it.

Both Aaron Whitehurst and Moffit connected people and problem solving while discussing the production and hiring of engineering problem solvers. Whitehurst recognized that influencing people to become problem-solvers and launching academic, industry, or government careers was part of his professional role. He specifically noted his expectation of producing engineers who can solve hard problems. For him, this meant that engineers should focus on "identifying what a research opportunity is" and "being able to evaluate the state of the art."

From a hiring perspective, Moffit reflected that in his recruitment efforts for chemical engineering PhD students his hiring decisions weighed more on one's problem solving skills than on their technical skills: "We didn't necessarily expect the thesis to have any direct applicability to what we were hiring." He suggested, however, that he was an anomaly in this hiring practice.

## Conservation

Respondents talked about the importance of engineering in core engineering knowledge and expectations, particularly "technical knowledge" (Terry Sherwood) and "being abreast of the current trends in the technology" (Shirley Thorne). Philip Hays described this technical expertise in great detail:

> They [engineering PhDs] need to have good analytical ability and to work with the appropriate level of mathematics. They need to have a good understanding of the physical principles involved, whether they're studying the thermal effects, or fluid flow, or whether they're studying, for example, in the microvalve we had to look at the magnetic field and calculate the forces generated. So you needed to understand the basic principles. And then you need to be able to put together these principles to solve an engineering problem of some significance.

Roland Bankston noted that foundational knowledge, or fundamentals, was the key to success for engineering PhD holders where they "understand the content of their field" and "the technical material of their field." Aaron Whitehurst professed:

> One characteristic is technical expertise, building up and understanding of some sophisticated … technical understanding. So that's kind of the classroom part if you will … being able to read literature and understand where the state of the art boundaries were, the technical expertise, the communication.

Both Whitehurst and Eric Dillard mentioned in great detail what they meant about engineering PhD holders' abilities to synthesize technical knowledge. Whitehurst said:

> One is an ability to be able to assess the state of the art and assess what is known and what isn't known in order to be able to judge select problems or

*judge whether the problems you're working on actually count as ... new research or if they're repeats of other things that are known they're not really research ... being able to assess ... what others are doing and put together a picture of what's the state of art of the field.*

Dillard's perspective connected closely to students and to his expectation of them as experts:

*One thing I tell my students is, you need to be the world's expert on this particular topic. You need to know more than me. By the time that they graduate I expect ... that we're working as equals and they're teaching me at least as much, if probably more, than I'm teaching them about the topics.*

*It's about understanding how to go beyond what you see, and synthesizing different information, and putting it together in new ways, and being able to expand your horizons in different ways beyond ... the narrow confines of, 'I did this measurement and this is what I got.' 'Cause anyone can be taught to work in a lab and be a lab tech. That's not what a PhD should be.*

## So what?

Across the characteristics identified across respondents, the overarching message for engineering PhD holders related to demonstrating one's technical expertise, communicating that information appropriately across contexts, and embodying core engineering skills (e.g., having the ability to problem solve) simultaneously. Although 88 characteristics were identified by respondents, stewardship (See Chapter 3) overwhelmingly emerged as a highly rated characteristic by engineering PhD holders working in academia and industry. This means that regardless of context, an engineering PhD holders should possess characteristics that represent high standards of proficiency and excellence.

Stewardship as a characteristic extended beyond one's technical expertise. Knowing fundamentals, however, materialized as conservation and as generation such that demonstrating competence was a key aspect of conservation and asking the right research questions in one's field translated to generation. Generation also included the ability to identify problems and projects that needed to be worked on in the field using appropriate methods and processes to solve important problems. Transformation incorporated possessing good written and oral skills, executing standard norms of communication (e.g., making eye contact), breaking down complex ideas for appropriate audiences (transformation), and translating technical knowledge for nonengineers.

The most highly occurring characteristics that were not stewardship included persistence, problem solving skills, and having a good work ethic. Persistence meant not being dissuaded or discouraged by one's research and failures and redirecting one's work as needed. Problem solving was a foundational characteristic for engineering PhD holders. since many innovations are not pre-packaged. As such, engineering PhD holders must determine how to move from visioning to executing their research. Problem solving also aligned closely with aspects of generation but differed in its focus on knowing *when* to change directions with a project. There is an expectation for engineering PhD holders to pivot at appropriate times. Similar to technical proficiency and communication skills, many respondents correlated technical proficiency and problem solving skills. Finally, work ethic connected to having drive or a fire to get things done and knowing when urgency was needed to execute tasks.

## Students

- Find opportunities to lead since an expectation of engineering PhD holders is to translate one's schedule and to offer guidance to others, especially to people without PhDs.
- Seek constructive criticism about your thinking, especially about research. If you are stuck on a problem, seek feedback about ways to move forward. Reflect on this progress for future challenges.

## All professionals

- Become comfortable with ambiguity since the role of an engineering PhD holder is to set vision and to determine when a research direction must change.
- Find ways to recover from failures quickly. Receive constructive feedback about ways to improve, and identify ways to pivot when negativity arises.
- Engage in lifelong learning that allows you to expand your technical competence and communication skills.

## Expectations

*I'm expected to be a very good teacher and explain things clearly, and care whether my students are learning or not ... I do a lot of prep work for my classes, and I think that helps me be a better teacher ... "Good teaching" with a focus on the individual student is ... the biggest expectation ... that my school places on me.*

**Sherrie Roberts, PhD, Assistant Professor**

Unlike characteristics, expectations are specific to an environment, meaning that the responses across sectors represent specific suggestions needed for engineering PhDs working in industry and academia. Top expectations for academics included teaching and research-related tasks, which are not surprises given the structure of higher education. In industry, expectations were more translational such that engineering PhD holders were expected to propel the successes of organizations where they worked (e.g., engaging in daily operations, solving technical problems, commercializing, communicating, working in teams, and engaging with constituents). Academia to industry respondents presented expectations closely aligned with the characteristics identified by academia to industry respondents earlier in this chapter. Industry to academia respondents mentioned teaching and research but also focused on grant writing as an expectation of engineering PhD holders.

## Academia respondents

## Teaching

Teaching was the primary expectation of academia respondents after earning a PhD. This is not surprising given the nature of higher education. When asked details about their teaching responsibilities, faculty did not speak solely about teaching but referred to the intersectional natures of their jobs (e.g., teaching and conducting research). The amount of time spent teaching across respondents also varied given their faculty roles (e.g., tenure-track faculty, lecturer, or administrator), their institution types (e.g., engineering specialty versus research intensive), their levels of teaching (i.e., undergraduate or graduate), and course types (e.g., capstone, laboratory, or lower- or upper-division).

Regardless of teaching variations, aspects of university teaching within engineering are somewhat constant. Among the responsibilities of engineering faculty respondents included teaching concepts in a classroom setting, advising students, holding office hours, guiding students in class, informing curricular innovations in a department or program, grading, creating homework, preparing lecture notes, meeting with students, developing new courses, preparing laboratories, and preparing students to enter the engineering workforce.

Sheryl Chambers, Catrina Benson, and Christopher Roe offered additional insights about how teaching aligned with their faculty roles. When asked about a typical work week, Chambers shared:

*I would spend time preparing for class .... working on lesson plans, learning objectives, activities to engage them in this objective, designing or choosing homework assignments, grading homework assignments or exams, and then also the interaction with the students in the class. So, the teaching in the class, meeting with the students after classes or during office hours to answer questions .... I'm expected to teach well. So I'm expected to work fairly independently to design high quality teaching tools, instruments, lesson plans.*

Benson spoke about her teaching process at an engineering specialty school and her preparation for teaching:

*So the evening hours are when I actually get to do all of those other things such as preparing for a new course, working on a grant, working on a paper, researching things on the web, writing labs, building labs. I actually bring home*

*equipment to do that kind of thing. If I'm doing something with robotics, prob-*
*ably programming the robot, most of that stuff happens on the weekend.*

Roe presented perspectives about teaching across levels and revealed how teaching is traditionally assessed in higher education (i.e., course evaluations):

*We want young faculty to teach both graduate and undergraduate level courses so they ... know they have to teach both. And also, before asking for a promotion they need to have created their own course. So, we're promoting the creation of new courses that are interesting to students.*

*... How do you evaluate teaching? Well, you want people to prepare well-informed notes and exams that have answer keys that are understandable ... and you look at the student evaluations which are very valuable even though students think that they're not ... in my department we are setting down as criteria to be evaluated.*

## Research-related tasks

Many faculty conducted research while teaching and engaging in service. Similar to previous responses about teaching, faculty did not have the luxury of solely working on research. Among the research-related tasks reported by respondents who worked in academia after earning a PhD included obtaining research funding to support themselves and graduate students; meeting with students or other researchers discussing existing and future projects; attending research group meetings; leading ongoing research projects; building research laboratories (i.e., personnel and equipment); grant writing; hiring; training and supervising students and post-doctoral researchers; reading papers; exploring ideas, engaging at regional and national levels; being aware of best practices and what others are exploring; staying abreast of new and innovative ideas in the field; attending conferences; reading and reviewing others' research papers; and reviewing proposals on panels.

Although respondents presented numerous examples of the intersections of their teaching, research, and service roles, Craig Daniels spoke primarily about her role as a research scientist with no expectation to teach:

*"I spend a lot of my time making sure that all the people who work in the lab, my post-docs, my graduate students, have everything that they need to be suc-cessful, they're getting good advice from me, and I'm spending time making*

*sure that they don't have anything to worry about but doing their work . . ..
make sure that they have money to go to conferences, and they have the software and computers, and the access to experimental stuff that they need
access to.*

*So, if you count the travel I probably average about a 60 hour workweek, and I
don't teach. So, it's very, very difficult in academia to be good with any mix of
teaching and research to be good at everything you need to be good at, you're
never done with your job. There's always something else you should be doing; you
should be writing your next paper, writing your next grant, preparing your lecture
notes, meeting with your students. There's always something else that you should
be doing over and above what you have time for. So my workweek is pretty frantic.*

*Well, in my environment I'm a scientist. So my job is to build my lab groups to
be the best it can be in ocular mechanics. My job is to write grants to keep
myself 100% funded, and my group 100% funded. Because I do research 100%
of the time, I'm doing the same things I did when I was a PhD student, I'm just
better at it. So, in a lot of ways the transition wasn't a transition. I went from
relying on other people to write grants and get me funding to building my
independent lab, writing my own grants, getting my own funding, and supervising my own students and post-docs."*

## Industry respondents

### Transformation

Presenting and speaking effectively were primary expectations of respondents
who have worked only in industry. Gennifer Rankin mentioned the importance of "knowing how to write clear, concise emails that people can understand and follow." Within industry, presentations are made to engineers in
other disciplines, nonengineers, bosses, customers, and upper management.
Poole lauded his ability to speak to people outside his technical area:

*"One of those things that I've discovered has made me particularly effective at
(Company) is that I can communicate with the mechanical engineers, and the
electrical engineers, or the data center technicians, or the CS (computer science)
people, or whatever because I can speak their language. The content of such presentations may include communication of fundamental concepts or processes."*

Referring to engineering PhD holders, Kimmel professed that "these
people will be capable of presenting ideas and technologies both at a very

deep dive level, but also at a higher level where things can be summarized, things can be explained to the laymen, or to high-level management in some cases to ... a very simplified form, and yet a form that communicates effectively."

## Teaching

An expectation in industry was teaching, although it differed from the traditional definition of teaching, which is an aspect of transformation. Roland Perkins explained, "They expect me to be able to teach the operators or the front line supervisors how to use that, use certain tools properly." Bradley Simmons elaborated on how he "scratched his itch" for teaching as an industry expert:

*I mentioned the academic interests that I had early on when I went to get my PhD and the real interest I had there is in teaching ... I've actually been able to scratch that itch for the last 20 plus years through the development of internal courses within the corporation here, and have taught a variety of engineering courses in the corporation again over the last 20 years.*

*The other piece of my job is I'm actually the Project Director for the development of a manufacturing engineering excellence curriculum where we are actually developing classes to improve the practice of engineering within the engineering function in (Company) and specifically within our factories. So I spend actually a lot of time on curriculum development, teaching, and deployment of classroom material as well as ... teaching others that are looking to understand and apply the techniques that we're pushing throughout the corporation.*

*The other piece of that, and this goes back to the curriculum development that I'm working on, is part of the expectations again as a result of the PhD and the technical depth that I'm expected to have is the ability to actually teach others how to develop, or build and develop knowledge almost like you would within a research program, and then turn that into a pack of solutions that won't have to be redone or problems that won't have to be resolved later simply because we didn't do a good job of developing the knowledge and then deploying it in the form of an effective solution.*

## Commercialization

Another expectation of many industry experts was to commercialize or patent their technical work. Julius Kimmel explained:

*I also am heavily involved in protecting the ideas and inventions that we create. And that's really an area that we call intellectual property management.*

*And that's dealing with our patents, trade secrets, copyrights, and some of the legal matters ... the non-disclosure agreements, consulting agreements, trade development agreements. And, I help to manage those sorts of things so that we can ... protect and control the intellectual property that we generate.*

## Solve technical problems

Industry respondents identified solving technical problems as a key aspect of their work. They were expected to see the bigger picture of a technical story and to dig deeply into problems. Although in-person and virtual meetings with local, national, and global constituents overwhelmingly occupied much of the time of the industry respondents, other daily engagement involved project management and tracking, staff reviews, budgeting, and email communication.

## Engage in day-to-day operations

Day-to-day operations in an industry environment involved working closely with customers, troubleshooting, and frequently communicating ways that problem solving occurred, including developing sound hypotheses, testing hypotheses, and running experiments. Julius Kimmel shared a scenario in which he solved problems:

*So much of what I work on is not just developing new things, it's solving problems with our plants and operations group where things have not turned out as planned, or there's been an escape, a product quality problem, first-pass yield problem. So we have to draw from all these experiences and make the decisions and solve the problems in addition to developing new things. So it's really a matter of drawing on all of these different experiences and fundamentals.*

Respondents often were not given the solutions to problems since what they were being asked to do had most likely never been done before. In many cases, a problem seemed nonsensical. Olgesby presented an example given to him right out of college: "When I joined (Company) I was assigned a project in the glass industry, the glass position, and the value was to develop a technique to handle glass without physically touching it." Additional challenges included the thinness of the glass and the potential for defects to occur during the glass drying process.

Although to a nonengineer it may have seemed impossible, engineering experts usually are not given options to say a problem is too hard or unsolvable. Possessing an engineering PhD brings with it an expectation that no matter how hard a problem is, engineers will find a way to solve it. Their job success depends on this ability to troubleshoot and to solve problems.

## Problem solving for teams

Although many industry professionals relied on their technical expertise to solve problems, several worked on teams to meet the needs of their organization. Benjamin Kinder reflected:

*I'm more or less expected to ... come up with these unique ... modeling capabilities to solve problems, challenging problems ... I support all of these different projects that we have within our group, when they hit a roadblock in terms of processes issues pertaining to my expertise ... If there are process challenges, I am expected to solve them.*

Bradley Simmons also recognized the need to problem solve with the team in his organization: "The expectation is that I will dive down on those [employees] that are most critical, or in some cases most in trouble, and are in need of guidance to insure that they stay on track."

Finally, Gary Braxton described his role as a project manager for teams and the problem solving and strategic thinking culture in which he worked:

*A great bulk of my work has been really more about organizing teams and running the project management side of things. So, I've apparently demonstrated reasonable success at that. So taking complex problems and reducing them into basically work streams and assignments for people to go off and do that then come together to create the common good. So, that's really where a lot of my work and really growing expertise has been ... I guess it's just in the day-to-day-the way we go about solving problems. There's a culture within this department that ... suited me very well, and it is a problem-solving kind of culture, and a strategic thinking kind of culture. So they're not at all afraid, in fact they encourage, people to think about what the right solution is, not what the expedient solution is.*

## Meeting with constituents

Respondents were expected to meet with a variety of stakeholders in their jobs globally and across the United States. These meetings often occurred virtually given time differences and other geographic factors. Stewart Oglesby described a global meeting in which he might engage:

*There would be parts of the team that I support that will not be in the United States ... they would probably be in Japan or China ... now it's daytime here, it's nighttime over there. And so sometimes you would be in four meetings with them doing presentations and going over data and trying to make sense of the data so that we can make the next move on what we will do; come up with another hypothesis; go to the lab; set up experiments.*

Nicholas Poole often arrived at work early to coordinate with individuals in various locations and to meet with others: "We've got data centers in various places so I wind up coordinating with them first thing in the morning. And then from there I will usually spend . . . about three to four hours a week in meetings . . . guiding my intern, helping him with problems he's having, keeping him focused on his projects . . . Kind of intern maintenance."

Gino Braxton shared what his meetings looked like in his position:

*There's a lot of conference calls and web meeting with people in Colorado Springs, and Memphis, and Orlando, and someplace else . . . We have a fairly diverse project that I'm also running. So, since the division project I've taken on the business lead for a couple of fairly significant cross-operating company initiatives. So that's what these conference calls come into play. So probably about a quarter of my workweek is spent with those.*

Meetings overwhelmingly consumed several industry respondents' workdays, however. Given the diversity of projects on which she worked, Arlene Petit estimated that she spent approximately 50% of her time in meetings with people in her lab and with people outside of her lab given the diversity of projects on which she worked. With the number of meetings that he must attend during the week and numerous daily tasks must complete, Bradley Simmons explained why he sometimes had to work beyond his 60 hour workweek:

*Office time is generally 8:00 to 6:00 with some amount of a few evenings a week or some time on the weekends, generally just to stay even with email communication and stuff like that, because so much of the core workday is spent in contact with and discussing things with others in the classes or the business and engineering leaders.*

## Academia to industry respondents

### Transformation

For academia to industry respondents, transformation as an expectation consisted of demonstrating technology to customers, possessing strong communication skills, teaching, sharing patents, and writing research papers. Blake Greiner explained what teaching looked like in an industry setting:

> Here we're viewed as subject matter experts. The rest of the company expects us to provide technical leadership. And so we need to get our work done through other people oftentimes. And to do that you want to be encouraging, you want to be facilitating, you want to help 'em, you want to be able to in a way point out the errors they're making. But at the end of the day what we want to do is to be able ... to get them to adopt our ideas as their own so that they have ownership for them. And so it often takes a lot of tact. It takes a lot of holding things in confidence. People will tell me things, and I hold them in confidence ... There's a certain amount of feedback that they could absorb material. That has to be monitored.

## Conservation

Conservation as a characteristic occurred when academia to industry respondents were knowledgeable and confident about their technical subject area. Blake Greiner described it as "what enables a person to do their job and keep their job." For him, this meant providing technical leadership to his company such that "if there's a technology that's emerging (and) could render a part of our business useless, I need to be on top of it."

## Operate as a domain expert

Academia to industry respondents referred to the expectation that they demonstrate technical competency and operate as a domain expert. Both Virgil Sharma and Ryan Zeigler admitted their discomfort serving as experts when they first entered their industry environments. Sharma uttered:

> "When I got to there I realized that ... I didn't feel comfortable in terms of getting the engineering experience that I really needed. And I found myself teaching courses and students in engineering without really having had the chance to practice."

Zeigler described his transition from professor to industry expert:

> "... while I had been an instructor you get this thing that your professors know all the answers, you know even when you get to be your PhD ... the advisory committee is the one to sign off and you still respect them. And now all of a sudden you've got this group of 30 people looking at you like you know all the answers. And it's like, "No I don't." So that was a very interesting transition.

*Because my default place is to be Professor Ryan. And, where I'm comfortable in understanding the details, and I tend to dive for the details, and a lot of people are put off by that. They see that as maybe intellectual arrogance. And at that point your message kinda' gets lost. And so, again I deal in a highly technical area. That is my job to be a technical expert. And yet, I have to communicate with people who know very little about my area to make business decisions based on that technical information. And that's a process I continue to work and learn at. That's part of the fact that you know I'm still learning and growing."*

## Industry to academia respondents

## Research

Meeting with graduate students, postdocs, and faculty collaborators on research projects, supervising graduate students and postdocs, working in a lab, leading and running research projects, thinking critically about research, reviewing literature, managing research labs, and writing proposals were the primary responsibilities of respondents who first worked in industry and then came to academia. Many of them emphasized the creation of an independent research program and of being responsible for the fiscal support of students and postdocs as placing great pressure on them as academics.

## Teaching

Teaching responsibilities mentioned by industry to academia respondents comprised teaching undergraduate students, teaching graduate students, teaching courses, preparing courses, doing problem sets, grading tests, directing students in class, and holding office hours. Reuben Moffit recalled the breath of his experiences teaching in industry and in academia:

*During my career at (Company), I did create and teach various courses along the way. Which is not quite like being in academia, but ... it was interesting as well. And so, then coming back to teach, which is, in general, much more on the technical basis. And around this time I was off teaching some managerial schools for future supervisors and things like that.*

## Grant writing and/or obtain funding

Several respondents declared the expectation for engineering PhD holders to write grants. Roland Bankston spoke about his initial frustration writing grants to obtain funding to support his graduate students and postdocs. Whitehurst identified grant writing as an opportunity to make decisions about the research he wanted to pursue in an effort to bring in the best students and work with them so they were "learning and becoming successful PhDs and producing research output on the way."

Both Eric Dillard and Shirley Thorne made connections between engineering and writing. Reflecting on his postdoctoral research experience and having the opportunity to write an internal proposal, Dillard confessed that during lab experiences with his students he writes all day, particularly proposals and papers. Thorne eloquently summarized the running expectation for engineers PhD holders:

> Being an engineer not only calls that you be an educator or mentor, but also a leader; to be someone who's able to receive research funding. So you have to be a writer. You have to be able to publish your work and to articulate your work to the larger community where they're able to understand it and hopefully use that information to better their life.

## So what?

Expectations were context specific, and as such, respondents offered detailed descriptions about what was expected of them as engineering PhD holders. Although the stewardship tenets of transformation and conservation emerged as expectations, several others that aligned with the everyday activities of engineers and mapped distinctly to academic or industry environments.

Similar to previous responses about communicating well with nontechnical audiences, respondents shared the importance of appropriate communication via email and others work platforms. Examples of this communication included teaching, research-related activities, and patenting such that engineering PhD holders became translators and facilitators for people in their work environments.

Conservation, operating as a domain expert, and solving technical problems aligned with the expectations that engineering PhD holders served as technical experts, especially in industry. Conservation involved staying abreast of the "state of the art" in one's field which served as a source of pride for many respondents who took their roles as engineering PhD holders quite seriously. For many PhD holders, this may be difficult since post-PhD, they are told they are experts but rarely have opportunities to execute this expertise outside of writing a dissertation and defending their thoughts immediately. As such, there could be disconnects between graduation and starting an entry-level position where one is a technical lead on a team. Solving technical problems was not a surprise expectations since engineers are expected to see the big picture and determine where their work fits within a larger project.

Commercialization is a dominant aspect of industry life for an engineer. Awareness of the translation of ideas into profit for a company is key for engineers engaged in innovations in their organizations.

Other general expectations for industry respondents were engaging in day-to-day operations and problem solving for teams, activities that extend beyond working in isolation. Day-to-day operations extended beyond technical boundaries and involved working closely with people or understanding business operations. Narrow definitions of engineering expertise were not beneficial to many companies that expected engineers to become integrated in the daily operations of that company. Serving as a problem solver on a team required that engineers answer questions that may not appear to have an immediate solution and that they answer questions in a way that allowed others to execute their assignments. In this way, engineers are leaders and do not have the option to say they don't know how to identify a solution to problems within their organizations.

For academicians, teaching and research were standard roles of respondents. Although many outside academia may perceive that faculty only teach, many respondents confirmed the intersectional nature of their jobs as teachers *and* researchers and the challenges that they often face trying to balance the numerous aspects of teaching with research expectations.

Many academicians also highlighted the expectation of grant writing and obtaining funding to support their research enterprises. They noted the complexity of grant writing such that they were expected to identify original research, to write about their proposed research ideas, and to recruit, hire, and manage students and other personnel to conduct their research. This expectation proved to be overwhelming for many and surprising to others who were attracted to higher education positions for a primary reason (e.g., teaching).

## Students

- If you are interested in becoming an academic, engage in activities that introduce you to teaching and ways to create and manage a research enterprise. Talk to professors who have been identified as successful teachers, researchers, and mentors so you can develop your professional development plan as an academic.
- If you are interested in becoming an industry professional, identify an industry mentor with an engineering PhD to discuss what the everyday expectations are for engineering professionals in your discipline or area of expertise. Start early in mapping activities that will prepare you for entering industry as a leader and problem solver.

## All professionals

- Engage in courses and professional development activities that extend beyond your technical expertise. This may include grant writing, project management, leadership, or public speaking, since the engineering PhD is only one aspect of expertise.
- Develop a plan to continue development of your expertise. If there are emerging trends in your field, determine how you will engage with people who can push you to a higher level of expertise in that emerging area. Ask your supervisor and colleagues for suggestions and for nominations to participate in advancement opportunities.

## Reference

Golde, C.M., & Walker, G.E., 2006. Envisioning the future of doctoral education: Preparing stewards of the discipline, Carnegie essays on the doctorate. Jossey-Bass, San Francisco, CA.

# PART IV

# How Do You Maximize an Engineering PhD?

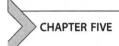

# Challenges during transitions and in doctoral education

*How do you go about coming up with an idea and finding somebody to fund it? How do you write a proposal that will read well? How do you put a budget together? How do you put together a project plan that supports your budget? How do you sell your ideas to a funding agency to build the research program?*

**Ryan Ziegler, PhD, Engineering Technical Steward**

Ryan Ziegler asked questions that addressed some of the challenges facing engineering PhD holders who are expected to build a research enterprise. He and other respondents shared candid stories about areas of potential improvement for engineering PhD holders working in academia and industry.

Two interview questions were combined to summarize the challenges respondents faced after earning their PhDs. One focused on transitions and the other involved doctoral education. Interviewers asked respondents to discuss the moves they made in their careers and how those moves occurred, along with the ways that they were or were not comfortable during these transitions. Respondents spoke candidly about their perceptions of their experiences transitioning from their engineering PhD programs to work or position changes within their working environments as engineering PhD holders. Specifically, respondents focused on three transitional aspects: (1) any job changes after graduating with an engineering PhD; (2) personal and professional reasons for transitions; and (3) respondents' degree of comfort with their transitions. The reasons for post PhD job moves included moving across organizations or to positions within the same organization, as well as promotions within an organization. Working on various projects within a position did not count as a job move. Transitions were classified as easy, difficult, or indifferent (i.e., not particularly easy or difficult).

For doctoral education, respondents were asked, "Do you think that during your engineering doctoral studies you obtained the skills to do your current job? Why or why not?" For each stewardship question,

*Demystifying the Engineering PhD.*
DOI: https://doi.org/10.1016/B978-0-12-801593-3.00005-0

respondents also were asked if their doctoral education prepared them to engage in generation, conservation, or transformation. Responses were combined and presented across four sectors.

## Academia respondents

Many of the challenges faced by academia respondents after earning a PhD involved the politics of academia, research enterprise creation and execution, and administrative responsibilities. Politics included learning the norms of academia. Creating a research enterprise involved developing lab policies, running a laboratory, hiring graduate students, and securing external grant funding. Finally, the administrative aspects of academic life pertained to learning how to lead efforts previously run by engineering PhD holders' research advisors, taking care of the needs of student researchers and post-docs, and managing general administrative duties. For some faculty, simultaneously teaching and transitioning from the role of colleague to boss proved difficult.

### Becoming the boss

Moving from the role of student to supervisor, manager, and leader was not easy for many respondents working in academia. Craig Daniels admitted:

> Probably the most difficult part of the transition is learning how to be a professional ... learning how manage your own situation and how to control, as best you can, your situation around you. So, sort of the biggest transition I've had probably is on the personnel front, trying to come up with policies that I think aren't too abusive but that still are reflective of the reality that ... there are two careers to be built in any relationship; the supervisor's career and the graduate student or post-doc's career .... the hardest transition is learning how, going from being a PhD student where you have somebody who's always looking out for you, always trying to make sure that you can be efficient and that you don't have any barriers to do your research. You become the person ... whose job it is when you start running your own lab ... you become the person whose job it is to remove those barriers for other people who are working for you.

### Learning academic politics

Another area of difficulty for academia respondents was awareness of and engagement with the academy's political landscape. As graduate students, many respondents were protected from the behind-the-scenes politics and practices that are commonplace in the academy. Stephanie Stahl alluded to gender discrepancies among faculty:

*You don't always get a good sense of how the political environment in academia works. That's one of those things actually that I've ... been learning ... there's some really significant gender issues that go along with that in terms of ... how people are recommended for awards and those kinds of things.*

Craig Daniels expounded on what it takes to learn the do's and don'ts of academia and how to affect change in an organization:

*When you need the policy changed, or you need something, you're trying to recruit someone, you want to affect change in your organization, there's certain ways to do that and you don't learn how to do that in graduate school .... The most uncomfortable part of that transition is learning, the hard way, how to make sure that you can get done what you need to do ... when I'm going to need a policy changed ... there are certain ways to go about that that are very effective and other ways that aren't. And you don't learn those things except through experience.*

## Writing grants

Responses about transitions and doctoral education both referenced limited grant writing experience and having little to no experience seeking and securing funding. Although George Murray, Catrina Benson, and Sheryl Chambers were exposed to grant writing as graduate students, they believed that this exposure was insufficient preparation for grant writing as faculty. Murray noted his shortcoming as not having "had a lot of experience in writing proposals as a graduate student although I was able to get some examples of successful and unsuccessful proposals from my PhD advisor before I left." Benson recalled:

*I don't feel I was prepared to write a proposal, or even really research papers, or direct graduate students, or run a research lab .... as a grad student ... we would either write the papers or help our advisor write the paper. He took care of all the grants. If he told us to write a paragraph for a grant we would write the paragraph, but we were never really involved in budgeting ... figuring out all of the kind of little nuances like someone like the NSF would want, like broader impacts, intellectual merit, etcetera .... I was flying blind when it came to all of that.*

She admitted that she did not comprehend the steps to execute the grant despite other positive skills she possessed as a graduate student:

*One reason I would say it didn't prepare me is because I never got to that high level but because I have pretty good organization skills ...I could do it if I had to. But as far as just being able to do the research and understand it ... steps in order ... develop a hypothesis, test it, publish it, get it done, and not even probably write a grant, I don't think I was totally prepared for that coming out of grad school.*

Like Benson, Chambers reflected on her lack of preparation and discomfort writing grants:

*I had limited practice doing any sort of grant writing as a graduate student. There was one course where we wrote a mock NSF proposal ... it was one experience and ... I didn't get a lot of practice with that. I didn't have a lot of confidence in my ability to generate creative ideas and make arguments to back those ideas up ... I didn't know a lot about the mechanics of the process about getting ... letters of support, timelines for getting other people on board.*

Stahl summarized why grant writing presents itself as a problem for many engineering PhD holders:

*When you go to graduate school ... you're expected to focus on a specific research problem; work very hard in the lab on it; and, write papers ... You don't get a lot of experience writing grants. So it's one of those funny things that ... you actually are in some ways ... not prepared to do ... you sort of do a lot of that learning along the way ... I would have benefitted from more guidance in how to write proposals as opposed to papers because it's a very different type of writing.*

Without grant writing experience, postdoctoral professionals and faculty continued to feel the impacts of limited grant writing experience. Mark Heard asserted that the career paths of many graduates are limited to postdoctoral research positions after earning their engineering PhDs. because they did not have "any established track record for bringing in money." Without an ability to write grants, many faculty limited their annual salary support by several months, especially during summer months when they are not given salary. Unfortunately, many faculty may not realize this as an expectation or limitation until they become faculty. Samantha Ayers admitted that she was "just now getting to the point where I'm starting to figure that out."

## Inadequate training to present effectively

Most academia respondents also expressed their inability to present and explain content to others outside of their technical areas of expertise after earning their PhDs. Both Sheryl Chambers and Christopher Roe discussed their difficulties communicating with non-academics. Roe explained, "Communicating to broader audiences and communicating with non-technical audiences- that's different ... I was not trained ... at the undergraduate or graduate level." Chambers reflected:

> Communicating with lay audiences, there wasn't a lot of training with that ... I did have some modeling of other professors who did things like speaking with policy makers. So I did understand that that was a part of what happened and maybe I knew that professors would give presentations for general audiences, but I didn't get a lot of training on doing that; on communicating with lay audiences.

Although Kevin Magee learned how to present while working in industry, he confessed that he lacked communication skills as a doctoral engineering student.

## Industry respondents

The difficult transitions of industry respondents differed greatly from academia respondents. Among the issues they found difficult was becoming a leader in a technical area, interpreting how one was performing in the workplace, traveling extensively for a job, determining what technical information to communicate and how to communicate technical information appropriately via email, working in a technical areas different from one's degree, learning how to work as a team more so than an individual, understanding corporate culture, and managing projects effectively.

### Working in technical areas different from one's degree

For many professionals, their engineering PhD area of expertise differs from the area in which they are hired. Nadine Vinson noted the challenge she continued to face working in a new technical area: "... when you're learning a new technical area I'm not quite sure you can really be a leader in it, but based on my previous experience, and the potential for the future, that was a promotion." Stewart Oglesby echoed this: "So, I joined the manufacturing, technology, and engineering division ... the challenges were ... what they do versus what I have studied." Gennifer Rankin also reflected upon this occurrence:

*In terms of the actual type of work I was doing, I was not so confident because the work that I'm doing now is actually totally different from what I did my grad work in. And so when I came into the company there was a pretty sharp learning curve because as far as actually coming in and doing the work, I had to ... learn everything from ground zero versus already having that particular background.*

## Assessing one's performance

Assessments of one's work proved to be an unexpected surprise for Arlene Petit and Nadine Vinson. Petit questioned annual performance appraisals in her reflection about the transition from graduate school to industry: "Every year we do performance appraisals, and I never did that in school, so how do you ... go through the performance appraisal process?" Vinson asserted that the evaluation of one's work performance was transparent in graduate school but not as straightforward in industry. When asked about her areas of discomfort, she explained:

*[I was] not comfortable with understanding how I was perceived, how my work was being perceived. When you're in grad school you get a grade for a course, your advisor kind of directs you on how your research is going, but you're not necessarily put up against other people from that standpoint. So, it was a little uncomfortable not knowing all the time where I stood as far as my performance.*

## Working with others versus working alone

Similarly, Bradley Simmons described his difficulty transitioning from working as an individual versus working as a member of a team. Fortunately, his company implemented mentoring and coaching practices to assist him. His responses highlighted gaps in training during graduate school:

*When I completed my PhD .... I was part of a larger research group, but we all worked as individuals ... we really didn't rely on each other a whole lot for anything that we did or needed to get done. And, when I moved into the industrial environment ... working collaboratively even in (the 1980s) was a way of life and something that I had to learn. I didn't really know how to do that and do it effectively. Were it not for ... mentorship and coaching, whatever that I had, coming into the organization that I joined here in (Company) I think it would have been very, very difficult for me. The other part that was a little more difficult ... was the change in attitude of doing everything for yourself which was certainly the way of life when I was in grad school ... you were expected to go out and lean on others ... independence was almost viewed as*

*being a bad way of approaching your job ... if you weren't leaning on the col-*
*lective expertise in the corporation be it a different division, a different part of*
*the company ... you actually were frowned upon ... it was shame on you if*
*you were trying to solve everything associated with a project yourself and not*
*relying on the others around you that had the knowledge at their fingertips*
*and you were expected to reach out to them and tap that knowledge. And I*
*contrast that with ... the PhD program where you know you were just*
*expected to dig it all up on your own and learn it yourself.*

## Inadequate training to present effectively

Industry respondents focused on presentation limitations from a practical, business perspective. A respondent's exposure depended on their doctoral advisor, the flexibility of that advisor, and opportunities presented to doctoral students within their graduate programs. Regarding communication, Nadine Vinson reflected, "I always continue to ask what really ... What is the broader sense? Why is this important? Help me understand where this is really ... practical." Benjamin Kinder mentioned this practicality and bottom line thinking also. He thought that although the ability to communicate in a practical way could be acquired in classes, the priorities of academia and industry differed. He explained:

*In academia your focus is solely on solving the technical problems and you're*
*presenting that to a bunch of professors, and they're also looking for that same*
*in depth technical detail. But on the other hand once you come in to the indus-*
*try that's not what everybody is looking for ... All that they're looking for is*
*how is it impacting them period. So, for me to translate all of that is always*
*hard. It's still hard sometimes ... I've taken a couple of classes ... I go ask for*
*a coaching from my manager as to how can we do this ... I'm a lot better*
*than where I was.*

Bradley Simmons also commented on industry's focus on translating technical content to nontechnical audiences. When asked if his doctoral education equipped him with the knowledge and skills to do his job, he replied:

*I would say no it didn't because we never talked about it, and we certainly*
*never had the opportunity to practice it ... the closest you came was being*
*able to take a significant body of research and distill it down to a 20-minute*
*technical talk, for example, at a national meeting or something like that. And*
*even then, you only got exposed to the technical side of trying to winnow*
*down what you had to fit a short time slot... You never had to worry about*
*presenting it to a non-technical audience, which is one of the things that you*
*would be confronted with once you came out in the industry. So very little*

*practice in that regard. And, in turn, it frankly becomes a skill that you have to acquire once you're out.*

Similarly to Kinder, Simmons has honed his communication skills since graduating with his PhD:

*I am not a charismatic communicator today by any stretch of the imagination but I am light years ahead of where I was coming out of my PhD program ... I can remember as we were getting to even go and present at a conference, it was the national team ... a lot of focus on getting the content right. Not a lot of focus on how the message itself was delivered. And, I had to learn about how best to deliver a message once I got out into the workforce. And to some extent still learning today ... The role that I'm in now I do, for example, more senior, more CEO to CEO staff level presentations than I was would have done ten years ago. And that's a little different communication style than it would have been if I was just speaking with the engineering directors around the corporation ... I wasn't even sensitive to coming out of school. I became sensitive to it as I grew in the workplace ... It's a skill that I still continue to have to hone.*

## Did not acquire specific technical knowledge

Although the engineering PhD holders acquired in-depth technical skills during their PhD programs, many still lacked several skills expected of them as engineering professionals working in industry. Stewart Oglesby recalled that his PhD studies didn't equip him to do his job directly. Gennifer Rankin acquired a job in a different field and therefore did not have "the knowledge to come in and really take off running." Julius Kimmel mentioned several of the specific areas of expertise in which he lacked but later learned on the job:

*Lacking statistics. And, only I had the DOE (design of experiments) background that I described through my class work through (PhD University), but I didn't have a lot of background in the usage of the tools that were available ... the computer programs, some of the tools that are out there, especially today. Now some of those tools weren't even in existence back then, but there were some, and I think I would've liked to have come in with a little more background there.*

## Academia to industry respondents

Areas of transition that proved to be difficult for respondents who worked in academia and then industry included teaching, running a research program, grant writing, managing a budget, and managing people.

## Teaching

Without prior teaching experience, Virgil Sharma and Peter Calloway highlighted their missing teaching experience as a barrier to success. Sharma noted his challenge entering academia, "I didn't feel comfortable in terms of getting the engineering experience that I really needed. And I found myself teaching courses and students in engineering without really having had the chance to practice." Calloway reflected, "That transition was difficult because a lot of new things that you'd never been trained for suddenly happened. You know, teaching ... I didn't do any teaching assistance or anything as a grad student."

## Managing a research program and people

The nuances of starting a research enterprise challenged Ryan Zeigler and Peter Calloway. Zeigler, who labeled the role of a faculty as an "entrepreneur boss," explained:

> I wasn't really prepared to be running my own research program because I hadn't seen how that was supposed to be done ... there was really the setting up of my own independent research program ... the business aspect ... at that point you become somebody's boss, or you hire a grad student- You're his boss. And now you feel responsible for them that you need to keep the funding coming so that they have a job. And again because there were older students, that one of my first grad students had a wife, a child, and I think their second child was born while he was my grad student. So there's a lot of responsibility there as an entrepreneur boss that was very uncomfortable for me.

Calloway referred to the difficulties of starting a research program in regards to fundraising, working with graduate students, teaching, and aligning with one's advisor:

> There are challenges there in terms of making your project work, and there's pressure ... But, in academia it depends on which position you have. I was at a Research 1 university, so I was expected to raise money, I was expected to have a lot of graduate students and teach, as well as serve on some committees and participate in any side projects that may come up ... The first challenge was ... that suddenly you're in charge of your research program. And you have to come up with new ideas that can get funding and that can attract grad students. But, at the same time, you don't want to just continue the same work you did ... because you don't want to compete with your advisor ... at

> *(University) it was really encouraged that you branch out on your own and show that you can discover new ideas on your own and not just be a continuation of what your advisor had done.*

Additionally, Calloway spoke about directing others being a challenge, particularly transitioning from managing students in academia to managing engineers in industry:

> *(The) third (challenge) is just direct my own program ... managing the students and motivating them to work harder and get their projects done. I think the bigger difficulty there ... was similar to going from the PhD to academia ... I didn't really have any specific training for the position that I was taking on. So, I went from managing graduate students to managing a group of engineers.*

## Did not obtain experience seeking and securing funding and/or grant writing

Blake Greiner and Ryan Zeigler referred to proposal writing as a need in engineering doctoral study. Greiner professed that engineering PhD holders "get very poor formal education" as grant writers. Zeigler presented several practical questions to guide a doctoral student in proposal writing:

> *How do you go about coming up with an idea and finding somebody to fund it? How do you write a proposal that will read well? How do you put a budget together? How do you put together a project plan that supports your budget? ... How do you sell your ideas to a funding agency to build the research program?*

## Industry to academia respondents

Industry to academia respondents mentioned fundraising, writing, technical knowledge, teaching, and limited presentation skills as challenges they faced.

### Fundraising

Industry to academia respondents primarily referred to fundraising and to writing as transitional challenges. Related to fundraising, Roland Bankston said:

> *The most frustrating thing about becoming a faculty member was fundraising. So that was because ... you have a startup package and you have about ...*

*three years to raise money basically. And if you're in a field that isn't a hot field then raising that money in the first three years can be very difficult even if you're very good because of fluctuations and the way awards are allocated ... So that was very stressful and that was something I didn't have to worry about as a grad student.*

## Writing

Both Randall Rice and Shirley Thorne spoke of writing challenges post-PhD. Rice noted:

*One of the things I was most uncomfortable about was that I didn't feel I got the proper training ... to carefully review literature and understand ... what are the pros and cons to the literature ... A lot of literature, especially in some of the fields I've been in ... there's a little hand waving going on and a little cherry picking in the data. And you've gotta' be able to sniff that out to be recognizing, "Are you really seeing the complete story? Or, are you only seeing part of the story?"*

Thorne reflected on her transition to a prestigious national laboratory:

*I was probably not comfortable transitioning from my PhD to (National Lab) ... in the area of being able to hold up to the (National Lab) standard .... In terms of publications, in terms of transitioning into that particular organization. And that took some time because I not only had to prove to myself, I had to prove to others that I was capable of that caliber of work which ultimately proved to be true.*

## Did not acquire specific technical knowledge

Both Eric Dillard and Randall Rice noted that given the specificity of the engineering PhD, they missed other aspects of doctoral preparation, particularly as it related to professional and technical development. Dillard acknowledged that some skills cannot be taught during the doctoral process but have to be learned over time. He also noted that working with a single research advisor often limits a doctoral student's technical and professional growth:

*That's not a fault of the particular PhD program ... to expect someone to come out of a PhD program necessarily being able to do that all that is a little too much. It takes some experience, some maturity ... So, no, (during the doctoral process) you're asked to do something fairly specific to ... be able to have those ... finishing skills, but within the context of that project ... For my current job, then you have to ... have a whole lot more than that ... You don't learn leadership skills necessarily. You don't learn how to go beyond different things.*

Rice also described not focusing of requisite skills that would benefit him after earning the PhD:

*I don't think my advisor ... gave me that opportunity to understand it [the complete story] ... I felt a little bit more of, "Okay, you can just go and do what you need to do, and get your PhD" instead of, "No, these are skills you need to focus on." Some of those skills came just because in the course of doing my project and my research project they were necessary to understand.*

## Decision to not engage in teaching

A couple of the industry to academia respondents had limited teaching experience prior to transitioning to their academic job. While Aaron Whitehurst learned it "on-the-job," Shirley Thorne was on a graduate research assistant who taught before and after her PhD program.

## Inadequate training to present effectively

Both Aaron Whitehurst and Eric Dillard listed limited communication training as professional challenges. Although Whitehurst garnered this training independently of his PhD, Dillard noted how preparation during the PhD aligned with expectations and tasks within a PhD program:

*When you look back, you see it's limited often in what you're asked to do. And so you're asked to ... do technical communication. You're going to write a paper, you get to write your dissertation, you're going to give a talk somewhere. You rarely are asked to do other things ... the different kinds of things I have to do now. I have to write project reports ... to NSF or some other agency, which is a different kind of communication. You have to write proposals, which are again completely different ... But that's typical ... get the experience of doing other things later as you're forced to do it.*

## So what?

Respondents highlighted numerous challenges they faced after earning their PhDs. These challenges emerged as they explored difficult transitions and doctoral-level experiences that might have been better for them and might have prepared them for their current jobs. Findings confirmed that despite the focus on technical competence, this competence is only one aspect that should be emphasized during PhD training.

Although engineering PhD holders engaged in higher education as students, most had no understanding of the complexities and nuances of higher education as engineering faculty. They were often unaware of academic politics, management, leadership, budgeting, fundraising, hiring, and daily operations of faculty life. To support their research enterprises, faculty needed to write grants, a skill that numerous respondents had to learn on the job. While many faculty advisors introduced respondents to general grant writing expectations, they did not engage actively in processes that ran the research laboratories in which they conducted their research. Similarly, although teaching was a big expectation of faculty, many respondents didn't report learning to teach as their greatest difficulty.

Industry respondents reported challenges that applied primarily to industry environments. They admitted that they often worked in areas that differed from their technical areas of expertise. As such, they had to adapt quickly to their new environments to demonstrate expertise, especially in areas with rapidly emerging innovations and technologies. Unlike higher education, industry appraises expertise differently from faculty advisors. As such, it was not always apparent how respondents were performing in their jobs.

Across all sectors, having inadequate training to present effectively emerged. Respondents noted distinct differences between communicating in academia versus industry and admitted they didn't know how to distinguish across those forms of communication. As such, many had to learn how to communicate orally and in writing in their current positions.

Other general challenges were not technical ones. Since the doctoral experience is a solitary one, there are often not opportunities for doctoral students to work on and to lead teams. If one is working in industry, however, teamwork is a required expectation. Although respondents earned PhDs, some were still not comfortable writing and engaging in the research process to produce quality scholarship. Respondents also noted variances in types of writing (e.g., proposals, articles) and needing guidance distinguishing between the writing types.

## Students

- Seek opportunities to lead in your research laboratory. Since advisors and principal investigators are busy, volunteer to assist with project management, research project reporting, strategic planning, and grant writing for your research group. Request feedback about the quality of your administrative efforts.

- If you want to be a faculty member, work on the development of your research group identity, which includes policies and procedures that will guide your research enterprise, hiring criteria, preferred methods of communication between you and your students and postdocs.
- Develop a mentoring team with people who can offer advice and feedback once you enter your workplace. Mentors should be available to answer questions in real time and should offer suggestions if unexpected issues arise on the job.

## Professionals

- Create a mentoring team that offers feedback in areas of need during your post-PhD journey.
- Share positive and realistic stories of professional life with your students so they understand real-life expectations for engineering PhD holders.
- Allow students to lead nontechnical efforts in a research group so they understand expectations of faculty.
- Practice tailoring communication in diverse ways to diverse audiences.

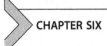

# CHAPTER SIX

# Recommendations

*The biggest thing is making sure that students are not hand held, that they are free — they're not told what to do, that they're in fact expected to figure out what to do on their own, and that they're given the freedom to make mistakes and correct those mistakes.But what that means is their project takes more time 'cause they spend more time correcting mistakes and less time making progress. . .There's a balance there. . . You don't want people to fail, but you also want them to learn how to be self-sufficient and find their own way because once they get out into the real world they're not going to have somebody sitting there telling them, "Here, do this. Do that." You're expected to be the one telling somebody else, "Here, do this. Do that." So if you've not developed any sense about what's likely to be right or wrong while you're a grad student- by making lots of mistakes about how not to do things, that's the quickest way to lead a PhD student to failure in post-graduate work.*

**Craig Daniels, Ph.D., Adjunct Assistant Professor**

*Demystifying the Engineering PhD.*
DOI: https://doi.org/10.1016/B978-0-12-801593-3.00006-2

This chapter presents recommendations from respondents and general recommendations for engineering doctoral education. The first part of the chapter presents recommendations from respondents, and the latter part of the chapter offers perspectives based on doctoral trends.

Although recommendations for the future of graduate engineering education differed across academia and industry, the most frequently occurring recommendations aligned with findings mentioned in previous chapters. Respondents were asked, "What can be done at the graduate level to ensure that students are acquiring the desired characteristics you mentioned earlier?" Tables 6.1 and 6.2 present combined high-level

**Table 6.1** Respondents' recommendations for engineering PhD students.

| | |
|---|---|
| *Advising* | • Develop a good student/advisor relationship |
| *Business acumen* | • Develop business skills (e.g., project management, running a research program) |
| *Connect with industry* | • Engage with non-engineering stakeholders<br>• Work on industrial problems with industry constraints |
| *Technical knowledge* | • Work on tough problems<br>• Cultivate a deeper understanding of technical knowledge |
| *Graduate program experiences* | • Select courses that align with desired and necessary characteristics<br>• Do a post-doc in a different department or field<br>• Participate in a summer internship outside the academy<br>• Participate in experiential activities |
| *Higher education changes* | • Align programmatic activities with institutional mission |
| *Professional skills* | • Gain leadership experience<br>• Participate in professional development activities<br>• Engage in mentoring relationships<br>• Network (i.e., build contacts with alumni or industry representatives)<br>• Develop organizational skills<br>• Take technical communication courses<br>• Develop good communication skills<br>• Learn to work independently<br>• Interact with diverse people<br>• Understand connections between engineering and society |
| *Research* | • Conduct research in a group<br>• Learn how to run a research program<br>• Obtain opportunities to conduct research<br>• Engage in interdisciplinary research/study<br>• Work on challenging problems |
| *Teaching and learning* | • Teach and/or mentor others<br>• Attend classes on teaching and/or<br>• preparing future scholars<br>• Learn how people learn<br>• Participate in discussion-based learning |
| *Working with people* | • Engage in group activities regularly |
| *Writing and presenting* | • Develop technical writing skills<br>• Pursue opportunities to present<br>• Write and receive feedback<br>• Publish in a peer-reviewed publication<br>• Find opportunities to write grants/funding proposals |

**Table 6.2** Respondents' recommendations for faculty, doctoral programs, and/or university administrators.

| | |
|---|---|
| *Advising* | • Guide students in solving an original problem<br>• Meet with students regularly to review their work<br>• Standardize mentorship and advising<br>• Do not isolate students from the realities of the work environment<br>• Expose students to faculty life<br>• Produce well-rounded students<br>• Develop a good student/advisor relationship |
| *Business acumen* | • Teach students about finances |
| *Connect with industry* | • Connect to industry (e.g., creating a survey & sending it via email)<br>• Expose students to industry<br>• Encourage students to communicate with industrial representatives via workshops, seminars, career fairs<br>• Acquire more industry experience<br>• Engage non-engineering stakeholders<br>• Work on industrial problems with industry constraints |
| *Technical knowledge* | • Cultivate a deeper understanding of technical knowledge<br>• Do not forgo teaching the fundamentals |
| *Graduate program experiences* | • Encourage students to study abroad for at least one semester<br>• Provide concrete instruction on professional ethics<br>• Set high expectations for passing PhD milestone exams<br>• Allow students to make mistakes<br>• Set a reasonable timeline for students to graduate |
| *Higher education changes* | • Change the reward system for faculty<br>• Empower faculty as they develop the next generation of scholars<br>• Control costs |
| *Professional skills* | • Expose students to new ideas<br>• Encourage students to critique their work |
| *Working with people* | • Promote interdisciplinary collaborations and communication |

recommendations for students and for faculty, doctoral programs, and university administrators, respectively.

In *academia*, the most prevalent recommendations aligned with teaching, technical writing, and presenting. *Industry* respondents also suggested technical writing skills and presenting as well as opportunities for universities to present doctoral students with more opportunities to engage with non-academic stakeholders during their doctoral work. *Academia to industry* respondents suggested that engineering PhD students work on graduate-level problems with industry and that universities facilitate exchanges with industry. Similar to academia and industry respondents, academia to industry respondents recommended that presentation skills be a major focus of doctoral student preparation. Finally, *industry to academia* respondents highlighted the importance of relationships between advisors and students, students' participation in professional development activities, and students' getting opportunities to present during their graduate school experiences.

## Expose children to the engineering PhD early

Pursuing an engineering PhD requires the collective efforts of parents, teachers, mentors, advisors, and numerous others years before a person earns that degree. Influences start as early as childhood, and recurring encouragement is needed when engineering students encounter academic challenges. There is no reason that pre-school and K–12 students should not know differences between a medical doctor and a professional who holds a PhD and that engineers who work in academia do more than teach. In the same way that STEM efforts are emphasized for elementary school students, efforts should be made to introduce students at all levels to PhD preparation before students enter graduate school. At the same time that students are learning about engineering and engineering subfields, they should differentiate what they will learn as engineers at Bachelor's, Master's, and PhD levels and should become aware of the engineering PhD as a viable option for their futures. Suggestions for parents and students are found below.

- *Parents* – Organize a tour of an engineering laboratory at a local university for your child. Search the engineering departments' websites, and identify potential topics and/or faculty research areas of interest. For example, if your child loves cereal, you might search a food or biological engineering website to connect with a faculty who researches grain. If the packaging of cereal is of interest, search an industrial engineering faculty's website to find a faculty member with a specialization in statistical quality control or manufacturing. Once you identify an area of interest, send an email to a professor asking if there might be an opportunity to tour a lab or if they can put you in contact with someone who coordinates lab tours. If the professor is not available, ask if a graduate or undergraduate student researcher might facilitate a tour or a conversation with an engineering researcher. Work with your child to prepare questions before the tour so the child can maximize the visit. After the visit, encourage your child to conduct a future study of the topic and reflect on how this might inform his future studies and career.

- *Students* — Push yourself to be a more independent thinker. If someone assigns you a STEM project (at any level), identify ways to expand aspects of that project. Obtaining a PhD requires an ability to envision a topic and to work with others to make that vision a reality. Realize that failure and conflict are natural elements of earning a PhD, so find ways to be comfortable being uncomfortable.

## Engage in conversations about the engineering PhD

Messaging about engineering, the PhD, and the engineering PhD needs to change. Unlike some legal and STEM professions that benefit from media exposure and from everyday awareness of their professions and how they contribute to society, engineering professionals often do not have such luxuries. Watch almost any television show, and you will see attorneys of all types (e.g., criminal law, divorce, district attorneys, public defenders, and prosecutors) and any kind of medical professional (e.g., surgeons, nurses, emergency room doctors, and psychiatrists). In addition, forensics has become increasingly popular given umpteen shows humanizing the medical profession (e.g., *Bones* and *CSI: Insert Name of City*) When engineers are portrayed, they are often viewed as stereotypical geeks lacking emotional intelligence and filling rigid stereotypes. At a minimum, media can inform people what the engineering PhD is, what it is not, and what people with engineering PhDs do.

- *Engineering PhD holders* — Write a blog, start a YouTube channel, create a social media account, or share infographics that communicate what you do. Photographs, graphics, and other visuals translate complex topics to people of all ages. When you produce academic or professional deliverables for your peers (e.g., a journal article), train yourself to produce a deliverable for people who may never enter your classroom or laboratory. There are numerous "how to's" on the web about ways to create any of these resources. The time it takes to communicate your work to new audiences is worth the payoff, because you are introducing potential scholars to topics and to a profession that might be of interest to them.

- *Media influencers* — A growing number of engineering PhD holders are sharing their work in public spaces. Begin by searching for them on social media since this is where you are most likely to hear their authentic voices, get a glimpse of their professional and personal stories, and get insights about ways that they contribute to society. Connect to these professionals for podcast segments, articles, and interviews to showcase their expertise to new audiences.

## Give the engineering PhD a face

For years, there has been a dearth of literature about the engineering PhD. As such, anecdotal information has informed the career trajectories of many engineering PhD holders. Although many future faculty may be aware of engineering faculty pathways (i.e., assistant professor to associate professor to full professor), details between those engineering faculty milestones vary and are often discussed in personal conversations. Given the privacy of industry, many engineering PhD holders also may not know what engineering PhD holders in industry do or how they contribute to corporate teams. With the increasing popularity of social media, blogging, and podcasts, however, engineering professionals are boldly sharing their good, bad, and ugly experiences as engineering PhD holders. As such, engineering PhD students are forming communities before they enter the workforce and are connecting to peers and virtual mentors outside of their universities and places of employment. Although earning a PhD in engineering is not for everyone, it is important to connect to people for whom the engineering PhD might be a viable career choice. Below are common questions and sample responses that might humanize the engineering PhD.

\* \* \*

*Inquisitive Iris*: When are you going to get a real job?

*PhD Holder*: Earning a graduate degree takes time, and part of my job is to conduct research in my engineering area of expertise. I work with a research advisor who guides me in my research. This training and the time that it takes to receive this training will prepare me to enter the workforce as an expert in (Area of Expertise).

\* \* \*

*Curious Carl*: What do you do everyday?

*PhD Holder*: (Explain a day or week in the life of an engineering PhD student. Although you may conduct research or teach, you also work as a team member and engage in daily operations that will prepare you to translate your research in ways that benefit society. Remember to use real-world analogies and examples that nontechnical people can understand. Encourage questions about your work, and respond as clearly as possible.)

\* \* \*

*Seeking Suzie*: Why were you in school so long?

*PhD Holder*: (Explain that a PhD is a terminal degree and that there are two levels that precede the PhD- the Bachelor's and the Master's degrees. Explain that to be an independent researcher or to create new knowledge in your engineering field, you are obtaining this final credential. If you choose to work in academia, the PhD allows you to teach others engineering fundamentals and to prepare others to conduct research as PhD students. If you work in industry, the PhD positions you as an expert who can engage with others outside your discipline to produce products that advance society.)

\* \* \*

*Questioning Quinn*: How does what you do relate to real life?

*PhD Holder*: (Inform the person questioning you that engineering is everywhere. Offer examples of your work and how it helps people. Use analogies if possible.)

## Identify exemplars in engineering graduate education

Although there are standard ways to assess engineering at the under-graduate level (i.e., ABET accreditation), there are no standard ways to assess engineering graduate education in the U.S. Assessment decisions are made at the discretion of graduate program faculty, which allows them autonomy in the development of their graduate students' experiences and in students' acquisition of technical knowledge and professional skills. Given a lack of standardization in graduate assessment, engineering graduate programs could benefit from the development and the implementation of assessments that extend beyond current milestones (e.g., dissertation qualifiers) and prepare students to begin their careers as engineering PhD holders with confidence and competence beginning with their first day on the job. Such assessments might emphasize both depth and breadth of experiences. Lessons may be learned from exemplary programs to achieve these goals.

- *Graduate Faculty and Committees*  — Questions to identify graduate engineering education exemplars include the following: What are the lessons learned from these programs? What assessments currently exist in these programs? How might these lessons translate across educational environments, cultures, and institution types with varying levels of resources (e.g., HBCUs, doctoral university, and research–intensive)? What assessments are needed to assess the skills expected of engineering PhD students? How might current and new assessments inform the experiences of engineering PhD students?
- *Policy Makers and Funding Agencies* — Consider resources might be created to promote engineering doctoral students' demonstration of technical and professional skills. For example, could a common repository be created across multiple to promote professional skills' development? Might efforts of exemplars be supported formally or at a greater level to provide resources to organizations that do not currently have resources to support their graduate students comprehensively? What lessons could be learned from undergraduate engineering education and translated to graduate education? Who might champion these efforts?

## Assess advisor/advisee relationships

Advising is a major aspect of life for engineering PhD holders. Although it may be assumed that advising comes naturally to faculty, the reality is that advising styles, experiences, and perspectives differ greatly. Negative aspects of advising might include mismatches between advisors and advisees or little to no faculty training to advise students. If advisors are not willing to admit that they need training, conflicts might arise. Without good advising, it may be up to students to obtain the skills they need to become successful during and after their PhD experiences.

Table 6.3 offers reflection questions for engineering PhD advisors and advisees. For advisors, share these questions with your current advisees

**Table 6.3** Reflection questions for engineering PhD advisors and advisees.

| Engineering PhD advisors | Engineering PhD advisees |
|---|---|
| • What is your advising style? | • What expectations do you have of your advisor? |
| • What expectations do you have of your advisees? | • What are your professional strengths? |
| • What are your advising strengths and weaknesses? | • What are your professional weaknesses? |
| • What is your work style? | • What is your work style? |
| • What is your leadership style? | • What would you like to do after earning your PhD? |
| • What are your preferred communication methods? | • How do you receive constructive feedback? |
| • How do you determine what advisees require of you? | • What are your preferred methods of communication? |
| • Where have most of your advisees obtained jobs? | • What do you hope to gain from your relationship with your advisor? |
| • How do you give feedback to your advisees? How often do you give this feedback? | • What kind of team member are you? |
| • How do your advisees develop professional skills (e.g., presenting, grant writing)? | |
| • What expectations do you have of your advisee by the end of their PhD experience? | |
| • How do you engage in one-on-one and group sessions with students? | |
| • How do you ensure that your advisees are prepared to succeed starting their first day on the job? | |

and compile the information to compare with your personal assessment. For advisees, create an interview protocol that you present to potential advisees prior to joining a research group.

## Connect coursework to engineering PhD pathways

Engineering PhD students often enter their programs wanting to focus on a particular aspect of the PhD experience. Experiences that differ from current ones need to be mapped out. An ultimate question is how doctoral programs might retain their credibility and focus on engineering fundamentals while preparing engineering PhD students in ways that are productive and aligned with students' ultimate career paths. In addition to standard preparation for graduate students, Table 6.4 offers suggestions of curricular, co-curricular, and/or extracurricular perspectives to engineering PhD holders pursuing a variety of paths. Suggestions are presented for engineering PhD holders who want to pursue academic or industry career paths post- engineering PhD. Academic paths focus primary on career development for teaching or research, and industry paths focus on career development for technical (i.e., engineering-focused) or nontechnical (e.g., leadership) paths.

## Conclusion

These recommendations represent a subset of suggestions for engineering PhD holders and other stakeholders. The diverse responses and respondents confirm that there is not a one-size-fits-all model for anyone considering an engineering PhD. The purpose of this chapter and other chapters in the book is to educate and to encourage people who think that the engineering PhD is unattainable and to provide clarity regarding possibly pathways to the engineering PhD. By sharing the successes and the failures of respondents, this book confirms that the PhD is attainable and that the people who earn their degrees have demonstrated persistence in their pursuits of technical excellence.

**Table 6.4** Suggested doctoral education activities depending on career paths.

| | Primary higher education focus | | Primary industry focus | |
| --- | --- | --- | --- | --- |
| | Teaching | Research | Technical | Nontechnical |
| **PhD experiences** | | | | |
| Become a teaching assistant | X | | | |
| Develop a course | X | | | |
| Teach a course | X | | | X |
| Create curricular materials | X | | | |
| Translate work to public | X | X | X | X |
| Develop teaching philosophy statement | X | | | |
| Write research proposal | | X | X | |
| Propose original research questions | | X | X | |
| Lead a research group meeting | | X | X | X |
| Mentor student researchers | | X | X | |
| Work on a research team | | X | X | X |
| Present to lay and technical audiences | X | X | X | X |
| Develop a research statement | | X | X | |
| Identify applications of research | | | X | X |
| Engage with nonengineers to achieve a goal | | | X | X |
| Participate in industry internship | | | X | X |
| **Curricular expectations** | | | | |
| Obtain a teaching certification | X | | | |
| Take communications course(s) | X | X | X | X |
| Takes business course(s) | | X | | X |
| Take policy course(s) | X | X | X | X |
| Take leadership course(s) | X | X | X | X |
| Gain exposure to commercialization and patenting | | | X | X |

## Suggested reading

Ahn, B., Cox, M. F., Zhu, J., & London, J. S. (2013). Investigating the attributes and expectations of engineering PhDs working in industry. In *2013 Proceedings of the frontiers in education conference*. Oklahoma City, OK.

Austin, A. E., Campa, H., Pfund, C., Gillan-Daniel, D. L., Mathieu, R., & Stoddart, J. (2009). Preparing STEM doctoral students for future faculty careers. *New Directions for Teaching and Learning, 2009*(117), 83–95.

Berdanier, C., Branch, S., & Cox, M. F. (2014). Survey analysis of engineering graduate students' perceptions of the skills necessary for career success in industry and academia. In *2014 Proceedings of the American Society for Engineering Education*. Indianapolis, Indiana.

Burt, B. A. (2019). Toward a theory of engineering professorial intentions: The role of research group experiences. *American Educational Research Journal, 56*(2), 289–332. Available from https://doi.org/10.3102/0002831218791467.

Cekic, O., Cox, M. F., & Zhu, J. (2010). Industry participation in the development of engineers as leaders in work environments. In *2010 Proceedings of the American Society for Engineering Education* (10 pages).

Cox, M. F., Adams, S. G., Zhu, J. (2011). Professional development for 21st century graduate students. In *Proceedings for the 2011 Australasian Association for Engineering Education Conference*.

Cox, M. F., Cekic, O., Branch, S., Chavela, R., Cawthorne, J., & Ahn, B. (2010). Ph.D.s in engineering: Getting them through the door and seeing them graduate- faculty and industry perspectives. In *2010 Proceedings of the American Society for Engineering Education* (7 pages).

Cox, M. F., London, J. S., Ahn, B., Zhu, J., Torres-Ayala, A. T., Frazier, S., & Cekic, O. (2011). Attributes of success for engineering Ph.D.s: Perspectives from academia and industry. In *Proceedings of the 2011 American Society for Engineering Education annual conference & exposition*. Vancouver, B. C., Canada.

Cox, M. F., Zhu, J., Ahn, B., London, J. S., Frazier, S., Torres-Ayala, A. T., Chavela, R. (2011). Choices for Ph.D.s in engineering: Analyses of career paths in academia and industry. In *2011 Proceedings of the American Society for Engineering Education* (10 pages).

Cox, M. F., Zhu, J., Ahn, B., Torres-Ayala, A., & Ramane, K. (2012). Recommendations for promoting desirable characteristics in engineering Ph.D.'s: Perspectives from industry and academia. In *2012 Proceedings of the American Society for Engineering Education, 2012*.

Crede, E., & Borrego, M. (2012). Learning in graduate engineering research groups of various sizes. *Journal of Engineering Education, 101*, 565–589.

Gamse, B., Espinosa, L., & Roy, R. (2013). *Essential competencies for interdisciplinary graduate training in IGERT* (pp. 1–109). Washington, DC: ABT.

Howell Smith, M. C. (2011). Factors that facilitate or inhibit interest of domestic students in the engineering PhD: A mixed methods study (Doctoral dissertation). Retrieved from University of Nebraska-Lincoln DigitalCommons.

Howell Smith, M. C., Garrett, A. L., Weissinger, E., Chandra, N. (2011). It's not what you think: A theory for understanding the lack of interest among domestic students in the engineering PhD. In *IEEE frontiers in education conference (FIE)*, 2011, p. S1F-1.

Lang, J., Cruse, S., McVey, F., & McMasters, J. (1999). Industry expectations of new engineers: A survey to assist curriculum designers. *Journal of Engineering Education, 88*(1), 43–51.

London, J., Cox, M. F., Ahn, B., Branch, S., Torres-Ayala, A., Zephirin, T., & Zhu, J. (2014). Motivations for pursuing an engineering Ph.D. and perceptions of its added value: A U.S.-based study. *International Journal of Doctoral Studies, 9*, 205–227.

McClurkin, J. D., Fitzpatrick, V., Cox, M. F., & Berdanier, C. (2014). Development of industry modules for engineers pursuing advanced degrees. In *2014 Proceedings of the American Society for Engineering Education*. Indianapolis, Indiana.

Nguyen, D. Q. (1998). The essential skills and attributes of an engineer: A comparative study of academics, industry personnel and engineering students. *Global Journal of Engineering Education*, 2(1), 65—75.

Nyquist, J. D., & Woodford, B. J. (2000). *Re-envisioning the Ph.D.: What concerns do we have?* Seattle, WA: Center for Instructional Development and Research.

Passow, H. J. (2007). What competencies should engineering programs emphasize? A meta-analysis of practitioners' opinions informs curricular design. In *Procceedings of the 3rd international CDIO conference*. Cambridge, MA.

Passow, H. J. (2012). Which ABET competencies do engineering graduates find most important in their work? *Journal of Engineering Education*, 101(1), 95—118.

Pilotte, M. K., Zadoks, R. I., & Cox, M. F. (2015). Harnessing engineering expertise in industry: Activating six sigma themes in a College/Industry Course Development Collaboration. In *2015 Proceedings of the ASEE annual conference & exposition* , Seattle, Washington.

Sageev, P., & Romanowski, C. J. (2001). A message from recent engineering graduates in the workplace: Results of a survey on technical communication skills. *Journal of Engineering Education*, 90(4), 685—698.

Stephan, P. E., Sumell, A. J., Black, G. C., & Adams, J. D. (2004). Doctoral education and economic development: The flow of new Ph.D.s to industry. *Economic Development Quarterly*, 18(2), 151—167.

Watson, J., & Lyons, J. (2011). Aligning academic preparation of engineering Ph.D. programs with the needs of industry. *International Journal of Engineering Education*, 27(6), 1394—1411.

Watson, J., & Lyons, J. (2012). Investigation of the work environment of engineering Ph. D.s in the United States. In *Proceedings of the 2012 American Society for Engineering Education annual conference & exposition*, San Antonio, TX.

Watson, J., White, C., & Lyons, J. (2010). Work in progress—creating industry ready Ph. D. graduates. In *Proceedings of the 40th ASEE/IEEE frontiers in education conference*, Washington, DC.

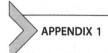

# Engineering PhD trends

*(1) What is the Doctor of Philosophy degree? What kinds of doctorates are conferred in engineering?*

The Doctor of Philosophy, or PhD, is a research-oriented degree. Within the field of engineering, potential engineering doctoral students have options to pursue one of two doctoral paths- a research-oriented one that results in the engineering PhD or a practice-focused path which leads to a Doctor of Engineering (EngD) degree (Friedland & Dorato, 1987). Several authors propose that alternatives to the PhD in engineering be created to account for engineering practice expectations in the field. While Friedland and Dorato (1987) champion the engineering PhD's coexistence with the EngD as a degree that engineering students obtain at the conclusion of their undergraduate engineering careers, Lyons (2000) identifies a professional master's level degree such as the Master of Engineering degree as a degree that can offer graduate students real-work engineering opportunites post bachelor's degree.

Kot and Hendel (2012) have conducted work exploring numerous types of doctoral degrees that may be conferred within engineering. They note that in addition to the doctor of philosophy degree, doctoral programs include professional doctorates, applied doctorates, practitioner doctorates, and clinical doctorates. Unlike the PhD, however, the purposes and definitions of these professional doctorates are not defined as clearly.

*(2) What is the difference between engineering PhD holders who work in academia versus industry?*

Within engineering, the term "practice" traditionally refers to industry environments, thereby leading to questions about whether there are different definitions of engineering practice in academic versus nonacademic environments. In recent years, Colleges and Schools of Engineering have begun to recognize the value of integrating practicing engineers within academic environments. With titles such as Clinical Professors or Professors of Practice, academia is identifying ways to blend perspectives of engineering research and practice. Nevertheless, questions remain about what engineering practice looks like in higher education environments.

Work tasks vary for engineering PhD holders. Within industry environments, many engineering PhD holders venture into management positions, while in academia, many professionals primarily teach or conduct research (Cox et al., 2013). This misalignment in the preparation of doctoral students for postgraduate careers outside of doctoral research warrants questions about ways to prepare engineering doctoral students for diverse careers- ones that require skills beyond those taught within their engineering PhD programs.

*(3) How are women represented among engineering PhD recipients?*

In their study, Nettles and Millett (2006) explored trends common among men and women pursuing PhDs in engineering. Aligned with national data, they found that more men pursue engineering PhDs than women across all educational levels (i.e., undergraduate, graduate, and postgraduate). They also noted that men pursuing engineering PhDs were more prolific publishers than women.

*(4) How do engineering PhD holders compare to other doctoral students?*

Nettles and Millett (2006) highlighted differences between doctoral students in engineering and doctoral students in nonengineering environments (e.g., humanities and social sciences) and identified trends that were common among engineering PhD students. Across disciplines, engineering PhD students reported the highest levels of satisfaction in their doctoral programs. They also made the fastest progress to degree completion across all disciplinary groups. In addition, social interactions between engineering faculty and PhD students were higher than interactions among faculty and PhD students in humanities and social sciences. Mentoring was also found to be highly correlated to degree completion for engineering students. Regarding peer interactions, however, interactions were found to be lower for students in engineering and education than in other disciplines. Finally, engineering PhD holders were more likely to be funded by research assistantships than teaching assistantships. Regarding career aspirations and career satisfaction, They noted that of the engineering PhD students in their study, 28% expected to become college university faculty or postdoctoral professionals, a number that is higher than the number of jobs available for engineering PhD graduates.

*(5) What are the career trajectories of engineering PhD holders?*

In a survey of engineering PhD students, Roach and Sauermann (2010) noted that the career trajectories of engineering doctoral students differ based on their preferences. Overall, however, the majority of engineering doctoral students think that the most attractive career options included working in an established firm, followed by working in academia, and then working in a startup. Doctoral students with preferences for earning higher salaries, accessibility to resources, and conducting applied research are more likely to work in established firms, while doctoral students who prefer responsibility are more likely to pursue employment in startups. Finally, students who have published more as doctoral students are more likely to pursue jobs in academia, which offers rewards such as professional autonomy and credibility within their communities more so than financial gain (Roach & Sauermann, 2010). Academic scientists were noted to have a "taste for science" (e.g., creating new research projects, publishing, and engaging with members of a technical community) (Roach & Sauermann, 2010). PhD students who have preferences for basic science research and the activities of the academic life are more likely to pursue academic careers versus careers in industry. Students noted, however, that one of the limitations of industrial research and development (R&D) work is potential limitation of disclosure of innovations (Roach & Sauermann, 2010).

## References

Cox, M. F., Zephirin, T., Sambamurthy, N., Ahn, B., London, J., Cekic, O., ... Zhu, J. (2013). Curriculum vitae analyses of engineering Ph.D.s working in academia and industry. *International Journal of Engineering Education, 29*, 1205–1221.

Friedland, B., & Dorato, P. (1987). A case for the doctor of engineering as a first professional degree. *Engineering Education, 77*(7–8), 707–713.

Kot, F. C., & Hendel, D. D. (2012). Emergence and growth of professional doctorates in the United States, United Kingdom, Canada, and Australia: A comparative analysis. *Studies in Higher Education, 37*(3), 345–364.

Lyons, W. C. (2000). US and international engineering education: A vision of engineering's future. *Journal of Professional Issues in Engineering Education and Practice, 126*(4), 152–155.

Nettles, M. T., & Millett, C. M. (2006). *Three magic letters: Getting to Ph.D.* Baltimore, MD: The Johns Hopkins University Press.

Roach, M., & Sauermann, H. (2010). A taste for science? PhD scientists' academic orientation and self-selection into research careers in industry. *Research Policy, 39*(3), 422–434.

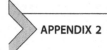

# Characteristics needed of engineering PhD holders (identified by all respondents)

- Able to apply a variety of tools to solve complex problems
- Able to interact with different people
- Able to justify your perspective
- Ambitious
- Analytical
- Assertive
- Balance theory and practice
- Be competent
- Be organized
- Be a public advocate
- Be quantitative
- Be willing to take risks, make mistakes during discovery
- Broad thinker
- Collaborate with others
- Confident
- Create and follow through a plan
- Creative
- Deeply analytical
- Demonstrate technical depth and breadth
- Detail-oriented (not research related)
- Document processes
- Entrepreneurial
- Experienced in organizing big problems
- Follow methodological and systematic procedure
- Follow through
- Get to the answer as fast as possible
- Global awareness
- Humble
- Imaginative (e.g., thinking "outside the box", being creative)

- Independent thinking
- Informed about current trends in technology
- Innovative
- Integrity
- Intelligent
- Interested in teaching
- Life-long learner (Never satisfied with a certain level of knowledge)
- Make predictions
- Mature
- Motivated by successful completion of challenging tasks
- Motivates others
- Network
- Open-minded
- Open to ambiguity
- Open to new cultures
- Organized
- Passionate about the subject
- Patient
- Persistent
- Personable
- Possess basic finance skills
- Possess passion for the field
- Possess both a deep and broad knowledge base/perspective
- Possess curiosity
- Possess integrity
- Possess interpersonal skills
- Possess leadership skills
- Practical
- Predict technical results
- Problem-solving skills
- Project management skills
- Put yourself in position of audience
- Read and cite literature correctly
- Research skills
- Resourceful
- Risk taker
- Self-directed
- Sociable
- Solve problems quickly

- Stewardship — Generation
- Stewardship — Conservation
- Stewardship — Transformation
- Take ownership of your future
- Translate findings into practice
- Translate your work in real world context
- Understand how to operate in a global environment
- Understand that there are different ways to tackle a problem
- Understand social implications
- Understand the big picture
- Understand the business aspects of an idea
- Understand the perspective of others
- Versatile
- Visionary
- Well-rounded
- Work ethic (related to the positive way of working or how you work (e.g., includes hard-working))

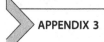

# Expectations needed of engineering PhD holders (identified by all respondents)

- Advising
- Affect policy
- Allocating fiscal resources
- Allocating resources (not fiscal)
- Always accessible
- Always connect via mobile devices
- Attend social events
- Be innovative
- Being accountable
- Be resourceful
- Building rapport
- Business skills
- Collaborate with diverse teams
- Collegiality
- Commercialize products
- Communicate with internal and external stakeholders
- Compete with colleagues for limited resources
- Conduct a careful literature review
- Create long-term plans for the business
- Create opportunities for students
- Design solutions
- Develop curriculum
- Develop the skills of the people you manage
- Document your work
- Economic development
- Educating students about solutions (faculty)
- Engage in business practices
- Engage in day-to-day operations
- Engage in international affairs

- Engage in policy-related activities
- Entrepreneurship
- Establish a lab environment with appropriate equipment
- Facilitating faculty success
- Fund people to conduct research on your behalf
- Gain a notable reputation in the field
- Grant writing and/or obtain funding
- Hiring or recruiting
- Independent thinker
- Liaise with industry
- Manage external entrepreneurial affairs
- Manage funds and/or make financial decisions
- Manage people (nontechnical)
- Meet high expectations
- Mentor
- Motivate others
- Multitask
- Network
- No difference in expectation from Bachelor's and/or Master's degree
- No expectation to publish
- No expectation to research
- No such thing as a "typical work week"
- Operate as a domain expert
- Outreach
- Participate in policy discussion and/or create policy
- Participate in setting up and running experiments
- Perform well with limited resources
- Possess adaptive expertise
- Possess leadership skills
- Prepare for your performance to be compared against your colleagues
- Problem solving (faculty)
- Professional development
- Provide technical support to other internal groups
- Publishing
- Quick learner
- Read policy reports and articles
- Receive feedback about your performance
- Recognize limitations in existing technology and empirical expressions
- Research

- Role model
- Saving costs
- See the "big picture"
- Service
- Solve non-technical problems
- Solve technical problems
- Stewardship — Conservation
- Stewardship — Generation
- Stewardship — Transformation
- Take initiative
- Teaching
- Translate theory into practice
- Travel
- Understand and meet customer's needs
- Understand the culture of the work environment
- Use modeling tools for decision making
- Visionary
- Work ethic
- Work in roles outside of traditional engineering
- Work on multiple projects simultaneously
- Work on open-ended problems
- Work-life balance
- Writing and reviewing papers

# Index

*Note*: Page numbers followed by "*f*" and "*t*" refer to figures and tables, respectively

Printed in the United States
By Bookmasters